The Child Within

Other books by Richard Butler

Behaviour and Rehabilitation: Behavioural Treatment for Long Stay Patients
(with Gerald Rosenthal)

Nocturnal Enuresis: Psychological Perspectives

Nocturnal Enuresis: The Child's Experience

Sports Psychology in Action

Sports Psychology in Performance (Editor)

The Child Within

The exploration of personal construct theory with young people

Richard J. Butler
and
David Green

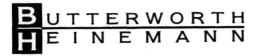

Butterworth-Heinemann
Linacre House, Jordan Hill, Oxford OX2 8DP
225 Wildwood Avenue, Woburn, MA 01801-2041
A division of Reed Educational and Professional Publishing Ltd

℞ A member of the Reed Elsevier plc group

OXFORD BOSTON JOHANNESBURG
MELBOURNE NEW DELHI SINGAPORE

First published 1998

British Library Cataloguing in Publication Data

A catalogue record for this book is available from the British Library

Library of Congress Cataloguing in Publication Data

A catalogue record for this book is available from the Library of Congress

ISBN 0 7506 2903 7

Typeset by Keytec Typesetting Ltd, Bridport, Dorset
Printed and bound in Great Britain by Biddles Ltd, Guildford and King's Lynn

Contents

Dedicated to our children

Joe, Gregory, Luke

Rachel, Katie and Joe

The authors

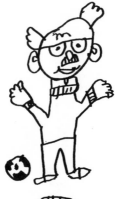

Richard J. Butler BSc, MSc, PhD
C Psychol, AFBPsS
Consultant Clinical Psychologist in Child
Health, Leeds Community and Mental
Health Services Trust, and Senior
Associate Lecturer, University of Leeds

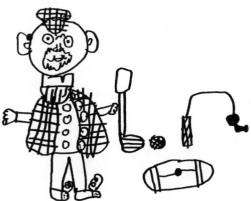

David Green BA, MSc, C Psychol, AFBPsS
Senior Lecturer in Clinical Psychology, University of Leeds, and
Honorary Consultant Clinical Psychologist in Child Health, St James's
University Hospital

(Illustrations by Luke Butler, aged 6)

What we take to be our knowledge of things
is actually only an opinion

(Plato)

Foreword

I was highly honoured to be invited to write a foreword to this book but I have to confess that this for me was a novel venture, never before having written one for another's book. Nonetheless I had dim recollections of other 'forewords' and presumed that this would provide an adequate briefing for this occasion. The nearer I got, however, to putting pen to paper and the greater the number of possible comments I had scribbled down as raw material, the more ignorant I felt as to what would be fitting for this particular text. How long? What kind of structure? What tone? I know of no 'scientific studies' on the writing of 'forewords', perhaps that subject does not qualify as suitable for investigation, so in default I decided to carry out a mini-project on the subject using the books on my own shelves as a normative sample. Looking at some twenty-five non-fiction texts, although there were prefaces in abundance, I came across only one 'foreword'. Are Personal Construct Psychology books any different in this regard? No, the proportion was just the same. So the result of asking this simple question is the remarkable outcome that the practice of eliciting 'forewords' is rather rare (p value approximately .05!). Why then such an invitation.

It seemed to me on reflection that a 'foreword' was not just a form of programme notes in advance, preparing the reader for what is to come. Rather it was a delicate way, at one and the same time, of (1) validating the writer of the 'foreword' by effectively saying 'You are just the person who really does know all about these matters', and (2) inviting validation of the book, and thereby its writers, by implicitly saying 'We offer something original and of value. Your recognition of this will confirm both us and the contents.' Under (1) the text itself offers validating messages by way of the generous quotations from my own writings and I take this opportunity of expressing my warm appreciation of the writers' generosity. My observations under (2) will come later and I can say in advance that they certainly will be validating but I hope will also point beyond. Be that as it may, I like both the delicacy and the implicit messages of the invitation.

As the title says, the theme of the book is *The Child Within* and is an account of the use of Personal Construct Psychology in resolving problems where a child is presented as the focus. The context within which this work is carried out is the hospital. This needs to be pointed out rather than taken for granted, since the resolution of comparable problems may take different forms when carried out in other contexts, e.g. child guidance clinics in the community, schools and social service departments. In particular, development in the uses of PCP may also take on different forms according to the context. It is a part of my credentials that my passport into professional practice as a psychologist was by way of the Maudsley Hospital, thereby giving me some notion of the hospital as a context but, more importantly, by being present at the birth of PCP in England. Although the odyssey of my developments of PCP in relation to child-focused problems started there nearly 40 years ago, it was continued in these other contexts eventually finding expression in Ravenette (1997) a text which in some ways parallels *The Child Within*.

I do not propose to go through the text chapter by chapter but rather to isolate some of its themes, both explicit and implicit, starting with the title itself. It is a matter of history that it is the adults who have spoken for, and on behalf of children. The essence of this book, mediated through its title, is that the child has his/her own individual meanings, and ways of making sense of themselves and their circumstances. Without finding ways of exploring these ways we are likely to fall seriously short in understanding those matters which lead to a referral. Even in some forms of 'therapy', designed to explore 'the child within', the meanings and interpretations are frequently alien to the child's implicit theories. The title points the way, in theory and in practice, to restoring the balance back from adult-centred to child-generated meanings, a most valuable corrective.

But the title does much more. Within Personal Construct Psychology the use of contrast suggests other, but related, issues consideration of which provide further balances against too one-pointed a stance. And these will probably be important when the child is presented as 'a problem'. Thus *The Child Within* suggests immediately a variety of constrasts: 'the world without', 'child versus peer group', or family, or parent, or school' each or any of which might well be important in understanding 'the problem' itself, in its broader perspectives, over and above the proper concern for 'the child within'.

My second theme is about theory. The value of theory lies in finding alternative ways of conceptualising phenomena such that they will be of greater value in dealing with those problems for which that theory is relevant. The grasp of a theory by the practitioner is measured by his/her skill in communicating its concepts in everyday language. The theory under consideration here is personal construct theory and the authors demonstrate their real mastery not only by communicating in the way I have just described, but also in demonstrating its value and application in the presentation of actual case material. The book is not for theorists but for practitioners, a matter of some moment since such books very rarely appear.

My third theme is that of context. As I said earlier, the work reported in this book was carried out in a hospital context. Therein lie potential hazards insofar as the communications are aimed as much to the outside world as to a hospital readership. A hospital has its own jargon which is taken for granted. 'Illness', 'disease', 'suffer', 'cure', 'treatment' and 'syndrome' are all common expressions in medically oriented contexts and may indeed be very proper in the case of physical disorders. They raise question marks, however, when they are carried over to the area covered by psychiatry, and child psychiatry in particular, since they reflect a style of thinking, knowing, and action which may be less appropriate in dealing with the vaguer complaints about children. Moreover the great attention given to finding 'diagnostic' labels to fit the child who has been referred, rather than the circumstances which the referral reflects, may carry the risk of looking in irrelevant directions if we are concerned with the circumstances as sensed by 'the child within'.

My final theme makes reference to the therapeutic work that was carried out with each of the cases. The writers demonstrate that a range of Kellian strategies are well within the possibilities of children despite the frequent argument that a high level of verbal ability is a necessary prerequisite. But I have a reservation about the word 'therapy'. I am aware that the expression has a long and honoured usage, yet implicitly it has the undertone that there is something wrong and it is the therapist's task to cure it. My own preference is to use the expression 'constructive intervention' which accurately reflects both the nature of the theoretical stance and the purpose of one's involvement in a case but without the framework of 'illness' and 'cure'.

It is, I think necessary to say all of these things, in order to make the point that the book is almost completely free of the hospital, or medical, atmosphere which might so easily have been communicated in the writing. I count this in itself to be a major triumph. I have to concede, however, what I consider to be one small fall from grace, but, and I say this somewhat cryptically, had the authors used the term 'dyslexia' in italics, I might have complimented them on a neat way of communicating doubt. Many, perhaps, might not agree with the validity of my observation.

All that I have written up to this point has been at a professional level but I plead licence, by way of concluding comments and at a personal level, to point to two special sources of delight. The first is to say how pleased I was to read short italicised quotations linking 'the text within' to 'thoughts from without' as elaborative subtitles for so many chapters.

My second source of delight is the reference to the TV detective Columbo and his 'naive' style of interviewing. Here I would also add my own favourite detective, G. K. Chesterton's Father Brown. And why? It seems to me that underlying all his successes is his implicit question 'Under what circumstances might this just make sense?', a truly Kellian thought.

It is my hope that this book will penetrate all those establishments where children are presented as cause for concern by those adults who carry responsibility for them.

Tom Ravenette
Epsom

(Ravenette, T. (1997) *Selected Papers: PCP and the Practice of an Educational Psychologist.* Farnborough: EPCA Publications.)

Chapter 1

Introduction

This creature called child might be the most elusive of all the creatures we have ever tried to understand (Epting 1988). Children do indeed pose a challenge. They can leave parents feeling exasperated, incompetent, culpable and teachers provoked, defensive and reproachful. Undoubtedly they can confound those to whom they are brought for help – doctors, therapists, psychologists, nurses, social workers and solicitors.

A major theme for this book is a search for ways to grasp the child's perspective. It aspires to make a difference: to lead to changes in professional practice, and more generally to the way adults approach and understand children.

Personal construct theory

Fundamentally our approach is guided by George Kelly's ideas, comprehensively elaborated in the theory of personal constructs (Kelly 1955). We do not intend at this stage to summarise the theory, as notable reviews are provided by Bannister and Fransella (1986) and Fransella (1995). Our aim is to explore the implications of the theory for understanding children's experiences. This chapter illuminates some of the major principles generated by the theory which have particular relevance for working with children. The chapters which follow take up these themes to examine childhood experiences in a broad array of contexts.

The underlying assumption

A root assumption underpinning personal construct theory is the notion of constructive alternativism, which essentially proposes that all our current perceptions, insights and understandings are open to question and reconsideration. For therapists engaged in the task of helping others change and reframe their experiences, such a premise could hardly be more heartening and optimistic. Change is always a possibility.

Kelly went so far as to conjecture that even the most obvious occurrences of everyday life might appear utterly transformed if we were inventive enough to construe the situation differently. We constantly create and recreate our own experience so that any aspect of our lives from the most momentous to the most mundane is open to potential reinterpretation. This splendidly liberating, but somewhat awesome, principle is as applicable to the child's understanding of self as it is to adults' attempts to understand children. Perhaps children need little convincing that there is always another avenue to be explored, another angle of attack to be considered. It is undoubtedly adults who are more likely to try and persuade themselves that they have discovered the 'real' meaning of events.

Such a sense of conviction is crucial to our capacity to act as effective decision-takers, but it has a downside. If in our analysis we have come to the conclusion that a particular phenomenon can be sensibly understood only in the terms of our favoured explanatory model, it is but a small step to believing that said phenomenon is 'nothing but' what we see in it. If the phenomenon in question is a child, pre-emptive construing of this nature can trap youngsters in the rigid categories that concerned adults have devised to help them with their problems (e.g. hyperactive, maladjusted, dyslexic). Kelly's message is a reminder that scientific construing, be it of the personal or the professional kind, is provisional in its nature. We formulate hypotheses to test. Certainly we live out our experiments, but always with a view to revising our theories in the light of experience.

The essential principles

If you want to know what's wrong, then ask
Kelly's infamous first principle. There are of course many ways of asking. A gathering convention amongst professional ranks is to ask by rote – swamping the individual with a host of prepared questions, either in questionnaire format or structured interview, so as to determine an appropriate category of 'abnormality'. Those adults in the position of caring for children often take a somewhat different approach – that of interrogation. How often is a customary 'Why?' met with a child's blank stare or 'Don't know'?

Both methodologies – rote questioning and interrogation – are however firmly resistant. They continue to be the adopted yardsticks by which children are understood. Perhaps the most extreme is where the questions themselves are presented in a standard format, such as in psychometric assessments of children's functioning. The results enticingly offer an understanding of the child, compared to others of their age, but may tempt us to consider the child exclusively in this way. Epting (1988) depicted the logical extension of such investigations by illustrating how many textbooks on child psychology remain silent on the topic of the child's psychology or personality, but offer 'intricate descriptions of cognitive development as if it were the same thing'.

Questioning of this sort seeks essentially to understand the child from the inquirer's frame of reference: is the child's behaviour abnormal?; does the child realise their actions are socially inappropriate?; is the child's cognitive capacity typical for his age? We might consider such approaches as ways of understanding children, but not as Ravenette (1977) cogently argued, as ways of understanding children's understanding. That requires us to understand young people from the inside looking out, rather than from the outside looking in.

Ravenette (1977) again invited us to consider that the basic tool of anyone charged with helping children solve problems and issues is the question, and that what is crucial for the professional is the capacity to 'invent better and better questions'. Ravenette elaborated 'better' to mean facilitative for the child and penetrating for the interviewer. Epting (1988) drove this message home by his insistence that any techniques and procedures we may adopt should 'always be in the service of a feasible portrayal of the human experience'.

The child is an architect of reality

Kelly (1955), and more lately, Ronen (1996) have suggested that children, like adults, do not merely react *to* the environment around them, but rather they act *on* it. They grapple to understand the world and their experiences in it. It is as if the world as given to all (reality) becomes represented to the child by the way he seeks to make sense of it. Events do not reveal meaning but, rather, how we represent the event to ourselves imposes meaning on the world.

Kelly's root metaphor of man the scientist, or in this context, the child as scientist, portrays the essence of the encounter. A child, like any other, cannot possess a copy or mirror image of reality, but rather a constructed version based on his experience of it. Kelly proposed the personal construct as his basic unit of analysis, as the means by which the individual accesses the world.

Construing is an act of discrimination whereby the child perceives similarities, themes and repetitions in the events before him. Once discriminations are formed the child is able to anticipate how events will unfold. As Mancuso and Adams-Webber (1982) described, anticipations are the schemata that are assembled to incorporate, integrate and assimilate incoming information. The child's understanding of events thus enables him to anticipate how future events might unfold, and in traditional scientific manner check out how well those anticipations helped the child make sense of the event.

The way we construe determines the way we act

This principle elaborates the anticipatory aspect of construing. Developing an understanding of events, through the process of construing, provides a hint of how things might go in the future. Such anticipatory inklings provide the basis of our actions.

As Ravenette (1977) has urged, however, our construing may lie at a low level of awareness. He further argued that an individual may not 'know' his constructs until a situation is provided whereby he is asked to produce them. People, according to Ravenette (1977), do not appeal to their construct systems in order to act, but rather, they *are* their construct systems. Thus all behaviour might be viewed as a testing out of the construct system. We test out our construing by behaving. Children's behaviour might therefore be seen as experimental. They test out their construing. They test out the boundaries, test how far they can go, and indeed test the patience of those who care for them.

If children's behaviour reflects their construing it may thus be possible to infer their experience or construing from their behaviour. Seeking to put ourselves non-judgementally into the 'child's shoes' can enhance our understanding of conceivable reasons for their actions. Our inferential tools, however, remain unsophisticated. Epting (1988) has urged for developments in useful procedures for what he called this 'reading behaviour backward'.

Children behave in particular ways because it makes sense to them

This principle emerges as a logical and related extension of the thesis that a child's behaviour reflects the way they construe. The notion that a child's behaviour makes sense to the individual no matter how bizarre, deviant, or self-defeating it may appear to the onlooker, is a pivotal theme arising from personal construct theory. The child's conduct would make sense if only it were possible to see the world through their eyes: a pretty sizeable task.

Gaining convincing access to a person's private perspective is far easier said than done, especially when children rarely have the awareness to deliver their understandings like the morning newspaper on the doormat, even if they had the inclination. None the less implicit in personal construct theory is the faith that there is always a potentially comprehensible relationship between an individual's actions and his constructions of the world.

Don Bannister's seminal work with individuals incarcerated on the long-stay wards of psychiatric institutions, who were diagnosed as suffering with schizophrenia, was perhaps the ultimate expression of this core assumption of the theory (Bannister 1962, 1963). Bannister sought to discover the personal sense in the construing of individuals deemed to be displaying classic thought disorder. He endeavoured to make an understandable link between their views of the world and their often seemingly bizarre behaviour. As a result of Bannister's investigations, he surmised that these patients employed such loose systems for understanding their social worlds that they could not reliably anticipate events. In consequence, their own actions seemed unpredictable and senseless to those around them.

In returning to the arena of childhood, it is precisely those children who most frustrate our efforts to help that we need to make the most conscious effort to understand. Otherwise we are tempted to give up and justify our ineffectiveness by resorting to hopeless explanations of human nature that locate responsibility firmly within the child, such as 'plain evil', 'lazy', 'thick as two short planks' and so on.

A preparedness to investigate the motives behind even the most deviant and dangerous activities of young people is not an intention to excuse. On the contrary, if public policy towards juvenile delinquency, for example, is not informed by proper scientific curiosity about the inner world of those who misbehave, it is unlikely to meet its stated aims. As surely as correct diagnosis needs to precede effective medical treatment, so an understanding of each individual child's experience should precede psychological intervention in their life.

There is nothing inherently wrong with labels. We need to categorise and make discriminations. Problems arise if the adhesive on our labels gets too sticky by half. What start as useful propositions end up as unalterable opinions as we slowly succumb to what Kelly described as the dread condition of 'hardening of the categories'! What we need is the psychological equivalent of those clever little yellow notelets that can be stuck on most surfaces to convey some helpful message, but are easily removed once they have fulfilled their purpose. The alternative may mean caging children for infinity in the pigeon-holes we have constructed for them.

Acknowledgement of individuality

Personal construct theory stresses how individuals differ from each other in how they perceive and interpret events. While we may confront common difficulties or share similar backgrounds, we invariably experience life uniquely. Kelly proposed a psychology that celebrated the singular way in which we appraise our existence. He recognised the different priorities individuals bring to bear in their personal analysis of the world around them, and appreciated the far-reaching implications of the interpretative framework we each evolve in our continuing efforts to make sense of our situation (Bannister and Fransella 1986).

That is not to deny that there are certain commonalities in our experience which are important to acknowledge. Personal construct theory is interested in similarities between the way a group of individuals view the world as opposed to similarities in the way a group of individuals are viewed by the world. For example, twins may look identical; their parents may choose to dress them in similar outfits; their friends and family may be unable to tell one from the other; and yet they will each have a singular opinion of the school they attend, the home they live in, and even the very business of being a twin. It is quite credible that when it comes to construing the world around them they might find they have more in common with another child than with their apparently identical twin. Rather than be surprised at this psychological divergence, families with twins tend to recognise the key role this 'personal' construing plays in the development of an autonomous sense of identity.

The respect for the uniqueness of individual experience that is enshrined in personal construct theory places a significant responsibility on adults wishing to use Kelly's ideas in their work with children. While at other times we may want to teach young people to use our language and appreciate our particular view of events, when following the personal construct tradition the job of the senior partner in the discussion is to get to grips with the children's perspectives. This means using their words, investigating their idiosyncratic theories, and respectfully checking to ensure we have properly understood what they intended to tell us; above all, never assuming we already know what we need to discover. Exploring the personal constructs of children is a serious undertaking.

Conclusion

The sceptical reader might by now have found himself reflecting that, if this personal construct theory is so optimistic and helpful, why haven't I heard of it before? This puzzlement might be further aggravated by the realisation that George Kelly, the author of the theory, first published his ideas as long ago as 1955 and has indeed been dead for over 30 years.

There is no mysterious tale of undiscovered manuscripts or arcane scholarship needed to explain our decision to write a book on personal construct theory in the late 1990s. Kelly, unlike several renowned American psychologists, did not market his ideas in the usual manner in which novel psychotherapies are sold to fellow professionals. He wrote at an abstract theoretical level, providing an integrated model of human understanding which could inform and enrich the practice of clinical psychology, education, child care, and human relationships in general.

Kelly did not, however, tend to be procedurally specific in describing quite how his ideas could best be translated into effective operation. It is unlikely that this omission from Kelly's writing was mere oversight on his part. Rather, he preferred to make those who chose to follow the personal construct way work out the implications of his ideas for themselves.

Within clinical psychology an increasing body of published research illustrates how productively Kelly's successors have taken up this challenge (Winter 1992). However, relatively few clinicians have explored the possibilities of using the personal construct approach with children. Our aim, therefore, in writing this book is to provide an accessible introduction to Kelly's theory as applied to the challenge of trying to help children in trouble. It is written in the expectation that the reader will have both an active interest in ideas and a pressing need to apply them.

The style and format of the book have been designed to mesh theory and practice by using a series of case studies to demonstrate how sometimes abstruse ideas can be translated into a workable intervention in a child's life. We have not however tried to produce a compendium of tried and tested recipes. To push the culinary metaphor a little further, we do not see ourselves as master chefs sharing our expertise. Instead, we aim to provide enough stimulus and structure to encourage interested readers to cook a little something up for themselves.

Chapter 2

The framework of personal construct theory

It has been suggested that George Kelly was somewhat ambivalent about the publication of his two volumes entitled *The Psychology of Personal Constructs*. Those who knew him personally, such as Don Bannister and Fay Fransella, felt that Kelly himself was unsure about the wisdom of seeking publication, although he remained passionately committed to his theory. Fransella (1995) discussed Kelly's reservations about publication, suggesting that he felt the psychological community in 1955 was not ready to accept the radical nature of his theory.

Fransella (1995) further noted that Kelly felt his theory would 'sink or swim in British waters', a prediction that was to be fascinatingly confirmed. Kelly's work remained largely overlooked and disregarded until Don Bannister stumbled across it on the dusty shelves of the University of London library, whilst searching for a psychological theory that made sense to him in his endeavours to pursue a PhD. Staying with the seafaring metaphor, it is appealing to wonder if Kelly's ideas would have remained sunk without trace had not Bannister conducted such a thorough trawl of the library shelves.

Bannister sought to test Kelly's ideas rigorously, particularly his principle that behaviour, however perplexing to an observer, represents the individual's search for meaning. Don Bannister chose the field of schizophrenic thought disorder. Rather than judge or diagnose the individual on the basis of his sometimes 'bizarre' behaviour, Bannister ventured to see the behaviour as an experiment. He wished to know what experiment the person was engaged in which made him behave in such a way.

Bannister's mode of enquiry was fundamentally based on the notion of understanding the person from the person's perspective, not seeking to fit him into a nosological category or a pet theory we may have about why others behave in certain ways. Bannister's impetus slowly gained momentum and workers in a range of professional settings began to test out the usefulness of the theory on issues pertinent to them.

Structure of personal construct theory

Kelly meticulously described the structure of his theory. According to Fransella (1995), this tallied with one aspect of his own psychological functioning which she described as his 'almost obsessive concern for detail'. Whether Kelly's own background as a physicist and mathematician contributed to this remains open to question. His immersion in methodology and precision as a scientist did, however, seem to influence his metaphorical notion of the person as a scientist. Kelly invited the clinician or therapist to regard the person 'as if' he were a scientist. As Fransella (1995) suggested, this leads us to consider that it is the person who 'conducts his or her own personal experiments to test out their construing of events' and the test we use is our own behaviour.

Formality of the theory

Kelly (1955) presented his theory in the form of a fundamental postulate and eleven corollaries (Bannister and Fransella 1986). The fundamental postulate states that *a person's processes are psychologically channelised by the ways in which he anticipates events*. Essentially Kelly was viewing the individual as striving for personal meaning. He argued that individuals grapple to understand their world. They perceive similarities and themes in the events before them, propose theories about such events, foster anticipations about the future and seek to test continually how much sense has been made of the world through their behaviour.

The world, it might seem, is composed of events. These are the objects or happenings with which we are continually faced. Kelly called them *elements*. They make up both the physical and psychological world within which we function. Quite how we make sense of the myriad of elements is the question Kelly was seeking to address in his formal description of the theory. He chose to outline this carefully with eleven corollaries which are summarised in *Fig. 2.1*.

A glimpse at a child's constructs

Robert was 10 years old when referred by his local general practitioner because of concerns about his 'hyperactive' behaviour. His school report told of Robert's difficulty in maintaining concentration and his mother expressed her anxieties about the way he was always on the go.

A short interview with Robert produced an understanding of how he perceived himself. He was invited to 'Tell me three ways that best

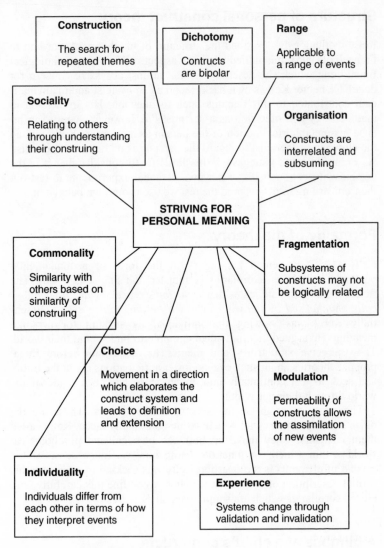

Fig. 2.1 A summary of Kelly's corollaries

describe the way you are', a credulous question, given the first interview. Robert had little difficulty in suggesting 'active', 'arty' and
'helpful', in that order. Perhaps, given the primacy of 'active', he too
construed himself, as others had labelled him, as possibly hyperactive.

'Active', 'arty' and 'helpful' can be considered as *emergent poles* of three constructs. Kelly described the emergent pole of a construct as *the one which embraces most of the immediately perceived context.* Asking Robert to describe the contrast to these poles by suggesting he might describe how someone *not* active, *not* arty, and *not* helpful might be, produced the *implicit* or contrasting pole of each construct. Robert suggested:

Active _____Boring
Arty _____Writer
Helpful _____Sit around and don't do anything

Kelly considered the building blocks of his theory to be constructs. His *dichotomy* corollary suggests that *a person's construction system is composed of a finite number of dichotomous constructs.* Robert had produced three on request but the likelihood was that he had many more (although Kelly stated a finite number) which enabled him to anticipate events before him.

Still with the three elicited constructs, Robert was invited to elaborate their meaning. Two questions pertaining to each construct often prove fruitful in furthering an understanding of a child's construing:

- 'Which end [of the two poles of the construct] would you prefer to be at?' This is marked with a **P**.
- 'When you are active [taking one pole of a construct] tell me three things that you are doing.' Alternatively the question can be phrased in terms of what other people do when they are being active.

The second question is called *pyramiding.* It seeks to understand the actions or behaviours that underpin the construct. It is extremely important with children to seek this understanding. Robert's responses to these questions were as follows:

Active _____Boring
  P
Playing games a lot
Running around
Playing sport

Arty _____Writing
  P
Building things
Drawing
Painting

Helpful _____Sit around doing nothing
  P
Tidy up
If someone is stuck, try and help
(Robert only provided two responses here)

Looking at Robert's responses there is a suggestion that rather than perceiving himself as hyperactive, he sees himself more of a boy of action. He prefers to be active, by which he means playing, tidying up and helping others, rather than be engaged at the contrast end of the constructs which imply boredom and sitting around doing nothing.

Constructs

Properties

The properties of a construct might be summarised as follows:

- An abstraction arising from an awareness of a similarity and a contrast between events. Robert had formulated this construction about himself by noticing repeated themes in the way he was behaving and contrasting this with the actions of others who did not behave in a similar way. Kelly summarised this in his *construction* corollary, which suggests *a person anticipates events by construing their replications*.
- Bipolar. The relationship between the two poles of a construct is one of contrast. Robert's three constructs contrast boring with active, writing with arty, and sitting around not doing anything with helpful.
- Arise out of an individual's personal experience and thus must be considered to be their own. Robert's constructs are his discriminations about the world. They are unique to him. Anyone else, in a similar situation, might have perceived different themes, similarities and contrasts.
- A means whereby an individual discriminates the events with which they come into contact. On meeting other children, Robert might construe them as active if they play sport, boring if they don't. He might also anticipate that those children he construes as active will also be interested in playing games. He might also consider, for example, when he comes across someone who tidies up, that he or she is helpful.

  Similarly, a child entering a library may carry a theory about books. This might lead such a child to browse a section from which they have found other books in the past to be a riveting read and ignore sections they anticipate hold books which were boring. The construct riveting—boring is operating to 'simplify' the environment. The same child might then employ a whole series of other discriminating constructs to help them decide which to borrow. Chapter 5 describes how intricate patterns of construing can be built up around subject areas through ever more elaborate discriminations, so that the individuals become expert or connoisseurs. Books might be considered to be physical elements. The same applies for psychological elements. Thus a child's previous contact with librarians might lead them to construe librarians as helpful, respecting of literature, quiet, intelligent and likely to wear glasses. If, however, the child hits upon one who grimly admonishes them for returning a book late, he or she might have to reconstrue their understanding of librarians.

- Imply that individuals do not appeal to their construct system in order to act, but that they *are* their construct system. Robert's notion of himself as helpful would move him towards someone he perceived was stuck. He wouldn't refer to his construing before acting. Ravenette (1977) has suggested that asking children to consider their means of construing, as Robert had been asked to do, might be the first time they are consciously aware of their means of construing. Much of a child's construing might therefore lie at a low level of awareness.

- The abstraction may have verbal markers. Robert was effortlessly able to provide verbal labels for the elicited constructs. However, constructs are foremost the discriminations we make, not the labels we attach to them. Kelly referred to 'unlabelled' constructs as *preverbal*, which are those which continue to be used even though the individual has no consistent word symbol. The construct may have emerged before the child had command of speech.

- Should a person take another person's verbal markers as a basis for a construct, he will invest it with his own personal meanings. Robert's notion of being active seemed categorically different from the pathological vision of activity that adults conferred upon him. Kelly's *individuality* corollary, which states that *persons differ from each other in their construction of events*, stresses the uniqueness of each person's construing, even where they may attach similar verbal labels to their discriminations. The contrast end of a construct helps define the meaning. Thus Robert contrasted active with boring, whereas many adults might perceive the contrast in terms of a lack of energy, liveliness and vigour.

Elements

Constructs, according to Kelly, are *convenient for the anticipation of a finite range of events only*. This is the *range* corollary. Robert's construct 'arty—writing' might well be useful in approaching school work, constructional play and homework, but perhaps less convenient in mending a puncture, fishing for sticklebacks or negotiating with his parents a raise in his pocket money. Would it matter a jot to Robert whether he addressed these activities as an artist or as a writer?

A construct thus has a range of convenience. It is best suited to a particular set of events or elements. The range might be very narrow or very wide. The range of a construct (and proliferation of new constructs) appears to narrow as an individual develops an expertise or connoisseurship in a particular area. Many children's constructs have a wide range of convenience. Thus 'boring' seems applicable to numerous events. Further, most children have an overarching construct of 'good—bad' which seems convenient to apply to almost every event.

Constructs of course are never fixed. They vary in terms of how permeable they are in accommodating new events or elements. Were Robert to try drama, cycling or fire setting and these were accommodated as either active or boring, then his construct would be considered permeable. Kelly encapsulated this idea in the *modulation* corollary, which states that *the variation in a person's construction system is limited by the permeability of the constructs within whose range of convenience the variants lie*. A construct is permeable if it admits new elements, and impermeable if it rejects elements on the basis of their newness.

Structure

Constructs rarely stand alone. Kelly suggested they are both interrelated and subsuming. He described this in the *organisation* corollary, which states that *each person characteristically evolves, for their convenience in anticipating events, a construction system embracing ordinal relationships between constructs*. There is a hint in the contrast poles of Robert's constructs – boring; sit around doing nothing – that these two constructs are closely aligned to one another. Were Robert to feel like tidying up (a behavioural expression of his helpfulness) after a game, the construct *active* might become more closely aligned to *helpful*. Thus for Robert helpful might come to imply active.

Kelly's notion of constructs subsuming other constructs is described in terms of superordinacy and subordinacy. Pyramiding is one way of elaborating subordinate constructs. Thus 'building things' for Robert is subordinate to being arty. When engaged in constructional tasks Robert would perceive himself as arty. One implies the other. Laddering is a way of eliciting superordinate constructs. This requires asking 'Why?' or 'How come?' the individual prefers one pole of a construct. Robert, with some hesitation, said he preferred to be active because 'If you're bored, you don't do much', arty because he didn't like writing a lot, and helpful because it was boring to sit around not doing anything. Robert had struggled to expand a more superordinate level. With children this is not unusual. Many children hold very permeable superordinate constructs often of a moral nature such as 'good—bad', so that most events are extrapolated as good or bad. Not being allowed an ice cream means the child perceives his mother as bad; a teacher who listens to the latest music is ace. With development emerges a more hierarchical structure, with psychological constructs such as Robert's active, arty and helpful sandwiched between subordinate behavioural notions and superordinate maxims.

Core constructs are those which essentially govern the person's view of himself. It might be postulated that the three constructs elicited from Robert are core. They fundamentally guide the way he thinks of himself and influence his behaviour.

As a construct system grows and evolves, subsystems of construing develop. Thus Robert might have a very different set of constructs when it comes to coping with his awkward and resentful brother. Helpfulness might not play any part in Robert's construing of such an event. Further, were Robert to take up train spotting, for example, he might discover a new set of constructs which serve this occasion better, including perhaps the benefit of 'sitting around doing nothing'. Kelly described this aspect of construing in the *fragmentation* corollary. This states that *a person may successively employ a variety of construction systems which are inferentially incompatible with each other.* Fascinatingly, a darts player may have a superordinate view of self as enumerate but can calculate the best way 'out' in nanoseconds

Comparison with others

Much diagnosis comes down to fitting a perception of the child's problem into a predetermined category of disorder. Much research too seeks to select participants on certain criteria with an assumption that a homogenous group is secured. Such procedures, argued Kelly, are crucially flawed. The *commonality* corollary suggests that *to the extent that one person employs a construction of experience which is similar to that employed by another, his or her processes are psychologically similar to those of the other person.*

Children are thus similar, not in terms of an 'outsiders' hypothesis, but in terms of their own typical ways of construing. Whatever the 'outside' consensus of Robert's hyperactivity, any similarity with other children similarly diagnosed is wide of the mark. An understanding of Robert's self construing gives this away. This is not to say that Robert cannot be understood as like other children. He might be considered similar to other children (or adults) who are guided by a sense of action, a wish to be involved and a distaste of boredom. Commonality is being 'like minded'.

Relationship with others

A central tenet of Kelly's theory, and one particularly salient for those in a profession designed to help others, is the notion of sociality. Kelly stated in the *sociality* corollary that *to the extent that one person construes the construction process of another they may play a role in a social process involving the other person*. This suggests that the success of any interaction with another person is based on the degree to which each person understands the other. Had we sought to understand Robert by way of a behaviour checklist, observation of his behaviour in class, an interview with his mother and a school report, a framework or 'external' description of his behaviour would have been achieved. This, however, would depict nothing of how Robert had considered his behaviour. The sociality corollary suggests an understanding of the other person's construing best fosters a relationship. It does not imply that the two individuals have similar construct systems, but that they are prepared to take a leap in understanding how each ticks. It may be that Robert's cat made a better stab at understanding him than adults who sought to impose a diagnostic framework upon his behaviour. His cat was able to detect when it was advisable to pester Robert for food and a stroke, and when, during his arty times, to leave well alone.

Movement

Bannister and Fransella (1986) described people as 'in business to anticipate events and if they do this by developing personal construct systems, then they will move in those directions which seem to make most sense, that is directions which seem to elaborate their construct system'. Thus it might be predicted that Robert would endeavour to be active, arty and helpful and seek to avoid boredom and writing. Kelly chose the *choice* corollary to define the direction of a person's movement. This states that *persons choose for themselves that alternative in a dichotomised construct through which they anticipate the greatest possibility for the elaboration of their system.* In electing to pursue a direction, 'being active' in Robert's case, a child is also clarifying and confirming a view of himself as active (Kelly called this *definition*). Thus each time Robert elects to play sport he asserts, in ever greater detail, his notion of himself as active. Additionally the choice, in Robert's case, to be active may lead to further elaboration of the system through what Kelly called *extension*. Should Robert be tempted to tackle his homework or clean out the rabbit hutch in his active way he may, as it were, be reaching out to increase the range of his construct system by exploring new areas. Thus, a choice to act in a certain way elaborates the construct by increased definition and possible extension.

Construct systems are continually developing and changing. They change in relation to the accuracy of the anticipations. Predictions will sometimes be correct. Robert might take to a new sport, such as rugby, in his active mode with an anticipation of enjoyment and evasion of boredom. His anticipations might prove correct and his notion of self as active and sporting would be validated. Sometimes, of course, predictions can be found wanting. Should Robert take up snooker, for example, with the same anticipation, his anticipations might be invalidated. Robert might thus attach snooker to the boring pole of the construct, active—boring. He might reconstrue snooker as not being a sport at all or redefine his notion of 'playing sport' as those activities which involve a degree of running around.

Kelly employed the *experience* corollary to describe the change in a construct system. This states that *a person's construction system varies as he successively construes the replication of events.* Any change necessarily involves a change in our self construing. Robert might have a greater sense of himself as sporting should he enjoy rugby and a more selective view of self as sporting were he to find snooker boring. Change within a person's construct system, Kelly argued, leads to the experience of emotion.

Emotions

Mildred McCoy (1977) sought to elaborate Kelly's original model of emotional experience, without undermining his expressed intention that the personal experience of emotion arises when the person is undergoing a change to the construct system. Some of McCoy's descriptions include the following:

Confidence
Confidence arises from the child's awareness of a goodness of fit between self and the anticipated event. Thus Robert might be confident

of doing well with constructional tasks given his liking and expertise in such areas, and equally confident of doing badly with a piece of writing, given his notion of self as not very good in this area. It is important to note that a sense of confidence is related to an anticipation of goodness of fit, not judgement about how well you might do. Thus children often show as forceful a demonstration of confidence for tasks they anticipate failing with 'I can't do that', as they do for tasks they anticipate succeeding in.

Happiness

Happiness is the validation of some aspect of self. Thus were Robert to successfully help someone who was stuck or complete a drawing to his satisfaction, this would validate his vision of self as respectively helpful and arty, and he would experience a sense of happiness.

Anxiety

Anxiety is the awareness that events with which the child is confronted lie outside the range of convenience of the construct system. Asked for the first time to roller skate, Robert might feel ill-equipped in terms of his construing to grasp this event. There may be further implications in that Robert might feel unsure about how potential failure will affect his construing of self. It is the inability to grasp the unknown which creates anxiety.

Threat

Threat arises from an awareness of imminent change in the construct system. This occurs where events force the child to reconstrue his vision of himself. Were Robert to find that he failed to succeed or enjoy his rugby ventures, he might be faced with a necessary revision of himself as an all-round sporting individual. His construing of self would be modified.

Guilt

Guilt arises from an awareness of dislodgement of the self from core construing. Guilt is experienced when we act in a way we would not have expected of ourselves. As with all emotional experiences described within personal construct theory, it is judgement free. An act of generosity by someone very careful with their money would engender guilt in the same way as someone on a diet eating a creamy chocolate cake. Robert might experience guilt were he to slob in front of the television. He would be acting in a way which contradicts what he would expect of himself.

Shame

Shame is the awareness of dislodgement of self from another person's construing of one's role. Shame is the result of behaving in a way that the child perceives is not expected of him or her. It involves an awareness of another person's construing, thus involving the sociality corollary, plus a sense that one's behaviour has not been as the other predicted. Thus Robert might experience shame were he to perceive that his mother expected him to put time aside before bed to improve his writing, but instead he chose to use this time to play games.

Anger

Anger arises from invalidation of construing, particularly where the construct system is in danger of collapse and there is no alternative way of viewing the situation. Thus Robert might become angry were he prevented from doing his arty tasks or discover that his attempts at art seemed always to lead to disasters.

Behaviour

Kelly described two behaviours, *hostility* and *aggression*, which also typically arise when an individual's construct system is under threat or requires elaboration. As with emotional experiences, Kelly also attempted to define these behaviours in terms of what is going on within the individual rather than in terms of other people's reactions to the child.

Hostility

Hostility is the effort to extort validational evidence in favour of a type of social prediction which has already been recognised as a failure. Hostility has thus a self preserving function. When invalidation of construing appears unremitting we may resort to rationalising, 'cooking the books' or deluding ourselves that our construing is correct. Were Robert to find his artwork marked constantly low by his teachers, and yet it remained important to him in construing himself as artistic, a hostile reaction might be to disregard the marks because the teacher 'doesn't like me'.

Aggression

Aggression is the active elaboration of one's perceptual field. It is the experience of pursuing a way of construing, actively experimenting to check the validity of our construing. Were Robert to throw himself into a new series of artistic endeavours in pursuing his notion of himself as arty, this would be construed as aggressive.

Therapeutic reconstruction

The philosophical heart of personal construct theory is constructive alternativism. Kelly pyramided this lofty ideal into its more playful and behavioural constituents. He described how the 'events we face today are subject to as great variety of constructions as our wits will enable us to contrive. This reminds us that all our present perceptions are open to question and reconsideration and it does broadly suggest that even the most obvious occurrences of everyday life might appear utterly transformed if we were inventive enough to construe them differently' (Kelly 1970).

Such a philosophical assumption suggests optimism about the potential for change. Individuals have endless capacity for altering the way they behave and construe themselves. The key notion in Kelly's abstraction is arguably that of the individuals 'inventiveness' to construe events differently. Without invention, creativity and imagination the individual is stuck.

The therapist, teacher, coach or parent wishing to help a child change or discover new ways of construing and behaving, might therefore valuably assist by fostering and supporting the child's inventiveness, finding creative ways to encourage the child to experiment, to discover the outcome of such testing and hopefully re-construe. Kelly viewed therapy as effective when it enabled an individual to undergo psychological reconstruction, so that he 'feels he has come alive' (Kelly 1980).

Reconstruction can take many forms. Winter (1992) has outlined some approaches which may be employed therapeutically to help an individual reconstrue.

Slot rattling or contrast reconstruction

A child might be invited to reverse his position along the pole of a construct. It transpired that in addition to not liking reading, Robert also struggled to master the written word. Slot rattling implies the rapid switching between the two poles of a construct, which in itself is not a stable form of change. A reformulation of the contrast pole is usually required. Contrast reconstruction might involve Robert elaborating the less favoured pole of his arty—writer construct. He might be asked to 'pyramid' writing to improve a definition of the behaviours involved in writing. He might be invited to observe and study the actions and attitudes of those children he perceives as being good at writing, and then try to experiment 'as if' he is a good writer.

A further technique employed by Tschudi (1977) invites the child to consider the advantages and disadvantages of both poles of a construct.

In Robert's case he might consider the advantages of being arty (being good at it; enjoying it) and the disadvantages of being a writer (failing; not liking it; boring) to explain a resistance to change. The reverse question of the advantages of writing (improve your learning) and disadvantages of being arty (Robert could think of none) might reveal Robert's impetus for changing. The implications of being better able to learn would provide a means of exploring Robert's desire to develop his writing ability.

The intention in Robert's case is not to 'switch' him from being arty to being good at writing but to help him elaborate the writer pole with a view to reformulating and hopefully delineating a new construct whereby he might construe himself as both arty and a writer, both constructs having a new contrast pole.

Employ another construct to the matters at hand

With only three constructs elicited from Robert the scope of employing another construct is somewhat limited. In practice a range of further constructs would be elicited. Nevertheless in an attempt to illustrate this type of reconstructive process, we might postulate a way Robert could elaborate his notion of self as a writer by drawing on another of his constructs. Robert might be asked to consider how someone who is active would tackle a writing project they did not like. The same question might be asked about how someone helpful might tackle writing. This creatively opens up ways of reconstruing writing. Robert might consider someone active would tackle a piece of writing with enthusiasm and someone helpful might reciprocally seek help off others when stuck. Robert could be invited to test out both ways of responding to future written work.

Increase the range of convenience of certain constructs

Staying with Robert's aversion for writing, increasing the range of convenience might involve testing the permeability of the construct pole. Thus enquiries about activities involving writing that Robert already undertakes, such as writing his Christmas list, might increase his awareness that writing is not necessarily tedious and followed by failure. Further, Robert might be introduced to new activities involving the written word such as wordsearch puzzles, writing jokes, keeping a diary of his best sporting moments or designing a new game, including instructions, as a means of increasing the implication that writing is fun, possible and an activity that can be completed successfully.

Test constructs for their predictive validity

This involves encouraging the child to experimentally test new constructs in everyday life. Thus Robert might be invited to act 'as if' he were enthusiastic, confident or studious when engaged in writing tasks. The intention is not to impose a form of construing on the child. Thus in asking Robert to tackle writing as if he were studious we are not aiming to transform him into being studious. The intention is rather to encourage a perception that change is possible, an observation of how this change is received by others and an awareness of what implications change has. Finally the success of any such intervention should be judged by how able it is to facilitate the child's understanding that they have the potential for change. They appreciate they have, in Kelly's terminology, the capacity for constructive alternativism.

Chapter 3

Communicating with children

At the heart of Kelly's theory of personal constructs is the insistence that if we are to understand a person's actions or assist them in resolving their problems, we must first make a determined effort to see the world through their eyes. Though we can chart through careful observation the objective challenges they face or infer through informed guesswork how they might feel in specific situations, we should never assume we know how any child is making sense of their particular experience. If we all essentially construct our own realities, we cannot begin to appreciate the psychological world of a young person unless we become aware not only of the raw objective facts of their life but also how they interpret their existence. Quite an undertaking!

Developing Kelly's first principle

Kelly devised a common-sense principle to guide enquiries. It was highlighted in Chapter 1 and suggests that 'If you want to know what's wrong with a child why not ask them? They might just tell you.'

A widespread reaction to such a suggestion might go something like 'What else would you do?' Kelly's seemingly banal piece of advice contains, however, a number of implications which may not be immediately obvious.

First there is the implicit reminder that the child is the expert on their own experience. No matter how stupid, immature, ill-mannered, or disinterested they may appear, each young person is the absolute world authority on themselves. They have expertise regarding themselves.

Secondly Kelly hoped to rehabilitate the question as a helpful way of discovering something about the inner world of children. Not all questions open up enquiry. Some questions can have a quite contrary effect, conveying the sense that the questioner already knows the right answer and is merely trying to trick or humiliate the person he is quizzing. 'Come on boy, we haven't got all day. Why did the Spanish Armada fail so manifestly to achieve its aims?', might reflect a conventional, if somewhat caustic, approach to accessing a child's knowledge.

'What possessed you to do such a thing?', is perhaps a more common form of inquiry when a child's behaviour is met by utter bemusement. Nonetheless when a question is posed because the questioner genuinely wants to discover something of which he is ignorant, and is prepared to listen intently to try and learn from the reply he receives, the process opens up possibilities. In contrast, when adults helpfully tell young people how they 'must' be feeling the likelihood is that the prospects of mutual exploration of meaning are killed in the egg.

Kelly's third lesson is a timely faith in the importance of 'keeping it simple'. Psychologists have a formidable repertoire of complex tools for investigating the human psyche – lengthy questionnaires, convoluted interpretations, galvanic skin-response monitors, sophisticated statistical packages and so on. Such an array of gadgetry is not required in order to listen carefully to what a young person is trying to say. Whisper it quietly, but there is a school of thought that says you may be better off without it.

Kelly's support for the simple principles of communicating with children does not mean we can discount matters of technique entirely. All of us, children included, have a wealth of implicit knowledge that we cannot easily articulate. We know more than we can say. Moreover those ideas to which we do have reasonable access are not neatly organised like some exemplary stamp collection, carefully indexed to help the casual observer find what he's after. Perhaps a more fitting analogy is the 'it's in here somewhere' frustration we encounter when trying to retrieve a mislaid letter from a desk strewn with a compost of correspondence! We need to develop some enabling strategies to allow children to begin to tell us their stories. Personal construct theory has fostered some fresh and inviting approaches in this respect.

Setting the scene

If children and young people are to be encouraged to reveal and explore their ideas about themselves it is important to create a climate in which such a typical reflection is experienced as a safe undertaking. Given our shared expectations that most of the questions adults ask children have right and wrong answers, we probably need to emphasise that, in our enquiries, there is no simple right way of making sense of events. We are after personal opinions. We would wish to respect the uniqueness of each individual's views and experience. Dare to be different might be the invitation to convey. Overall the enquirer's message is that he wants above all else to try and understand what the children are getting at – what they mean to say in their own terms.

It is a rare luxury for any person to be afforded the time and respect to feel properly understood by another. For an adult to pay such privileged attention to a child is perhaps an even more exceptional occurrence. We should therefore anticipate that our carefully crafted questions may initially be treated with suspicion. One way that adolescents, in particular, may be tempted to test out how convincingly an adult – be they teacher, therapist, or parent – plays this role of understanding investigator, is to 'con' or deliberately mislead this apparently concerned grown-up to see how they will react. The adult then faces a familiar dilemma. Do they accept as trustworthy some evident falsehood and run the risk of being dismissed as some easily-duped dunderhead not worthy of being taken seriously? Or, do they challenge the accuracy of the account the young person has provided and so stand accused of crass hypocrisy in claiming to respect the adolescent's opinions and then call him a liar in the next breath? Get out of that!

Kelly advocated that we try to set aside our fear of being deceived, and adopt what he termed a 'credulous' approach to the young people with whom we work. Believe what they tell us. Even if faced with what appear implausible accounts of events, the listener responds in good faith in the expectation that this exchange will ultimately make sense once the speaker's scheme of things is more fully understood. So, for example, a troubled school pupil who denies he has any learning problems may need to know that it is his view of events rather than his teacher's opinion which is going to be validated, before he can acknowledge his areas of difficulty.

When Peter Falk played the TV detective Columbo he seemed to convey just this sort of trusting bemusement as he scratched his head and asked suspects if they would kindly go through their stories 'one more time' so he could make sure he understood properly what they wanted to convey to him.

Ways of eliciting constructs

Traditional

Personal construct theory holds that individuals have a unique but limited set of discriminations which they use to define their experience. As outlined in Chapter 2, the discriminations are termed constructs. Constructs are considered to have two poles, opposite in meaning, that allow the individual to make sense of a restricted range of phenomena. So a construct such as 'diligent—lazy' might describe an attitude to work, but would, in all probability, not be relevant to a consideration of the different curry dishes on the menu of a favourite Indian restaurant, where 'blows your head off—mild as milk' would fit the bill much better.

Conversations with children might seek to discover which constructs they employ in relation to key issues in their lives. When learning to speak their language we aspire not just to use their words but also to grasp their meaning. Kelly devised a straightforward sorting system to elicit constructs relevant to particular concerns. This involved taking three elements, or events, such as the names of family members, subjects studied at school, or possible holiday destinations, and asking an individual 'in which way are two of these [people, subjects, places or whatever] the same and therefore different from the third?' This form of triadic questioning might elicit a reply like 'My mum and sister like to talk a lot but my grandad doesn't say much.'

Sometimes this three-way comparison proves conceptually difficult, especially for younger children, but inviting contrasts between a pair of elements is a less demanding request. Thus a child might be invited to consider how two elements compare, either in their similarity or difference. A child might perceive a similarity between themselves and a friend in terms of them both liking animals. This represents, then, one pole of a construct to do with respect for natural history. The contrast pole might emerge by inviting the child to describe someone who doesn't like animals. A child focusing on the difference between two elements such as sleeping in your own bed and staying overnight at a friend's house might perceive the difference in terms of sometimes being scared when waking up away from home. Means of discovering children's construing in these ways have been discussed by Salmon (1976) and Butler (1985).

Self descriptions

Perhaps a much simpler means of eliciting constructs is to ask the child to consider not three or even two elements, but just one. A favoured line of questioning suggested by Tom Ravenette (1977) is to ask the child to evaluate themselves as they think others see them.

- The child is asked, 'Who do you think knows you best of all?' A list of individuals significant to the child is built up from this. The list might include, in addition to family, friends, teachers and others, the child's pet, favourite cartoon figure, esteemed sporting hero and the child themselves.
- Taking the individuals from the list one at a time, the child is invited to describe themselves as they perceive others view them. They are asked, 'If I were to ask [e.g. your mother] to describe you, to tell me the three most important things he or she

could say about you, what *three* things would he or she say?' In metaphorically trying to stand in another person's shoes the child feels perhaps less apprehensive about describing him- or herself. However, given Kelly's notions about the individuality, uniqueness and ownership of constructs, the child in endeavouring to respond to this question is doing so by means of their own construct system.

- The contrast pole of each description can be sought by asking the child to describe someone who is not like the emerged pole.

Who are you?

This represents a direct request to the young person to say who he or she is. In Chapter 2 Robert was invited to respond to such an inquiry.

- The question runs along the following lines: 'If I were to ask you to tell me three things that best describe you, what would you say. Who are you?'
- After seeking the contrast pole to each description, each construct can be elaborated in various ways. The child can be asked which end they would prefer to be at. This indicates the degree to which the child is content or dissatisfied with him- or herself.
- The child might be invited, as Ravenette suggested, to describe what is important or special about the preferred end of a construct. This elaborates the personal meaning. It may also produce higher order or more superordinate constructs. If a child comes up with a series of physical constructs such as 'stocky', 'black hair' or 'spotty', such questioning about the importance of such descriptions for the child can lead to the emergence of more psychological constructs.
- Moving in the opposite direction, a child might be invited to describe the behavioural constituents of a construct through the process of pyramiding. This was undertaken with Robert in the preceding chapter, and essentially requires asking the child to describe what a person typically does when they are described by the construct. Thus an intricate elaboration of 'moody', for example, can be discerned by asking the child to describe what a person tends to do when they are being moody.

Tell me three things

Ravenette found another way of using the magic number 3 in eliciting children's constructs. The child is invited to express their view on events, situations and problems which are located onto an imagined other child. Thus a child is asked, 'Tell me three things about ... [e.g. the sort of girl who worries about going to school]'. This might be met with the following reply:

1. She doesn't like sums.
2. She loves her mummy.
3. She hasn't got any friends.

There is of course no magic about the number 3, nor any law about extracting a third construct if a youngster can easily produce only two. The purpose of the exercise is to pose a question in a form with which schoolchildren, in particular, will be familiar and to set a manageable challenge.

Self characterisation

Very often we are primarily interested in what children make of themselves (how they view themselves): compared with their views of other young people; compared with the person they would like to be; compared with the person they imagine their mum or dad would like them to be; and so on. Kelly devised an exercise termed self characterisation, which invites the young person to describe themselves as if a character in a play. Jackson (1987) provides a full account of this technique. The idea is that by writing in the third person an individual can step back from themselves a little and draw a pithy portrait of what they consider the essential elements of their personality. The only other instruction to the creator of a self characterisation is to write with an intimate and sympathetic understanding of your subject. Sometimes this simple framework helps people produce a candid and powerful précis of how they construe themselves. For example:

> Neil is 15-years-old and goes to the King's High School. He is taking GCSE examinations in June this year. He is shy and is always vulnerable and finds it very difficult to communicate and get over ideas and very often is lost for words and as a result is laughed at regularly. Neil finds it difficult to make friends and as he is vulnerable, he always makes mistakes when talking to a large group of people, e.g. in class discussions at school. The worst problem is getting across ideas, and instead he says stupid things.
> Neil is very shy and appears queer and he is also very boring. He appears upset and as a result he usually makes a fool of himself.

This account was written by a 15-year-old lad who evidently understood the task well enough, though significantly he elected to emphasise his perceived failings despite the invitation to be gentle on himself. He raised a series of constructs concerned with a sense of shyness, vulnerability and a difficulty in communicating. Neil also highlighted some implications of being like this, including being lost for words, saying stupid things and being laughed at.

Younger, or less able, informants sometimes struggle to grasp the 'official' format of the self characterisation. They may feel ill at ease with the artificiality of writing about themselves in the third person. Offering to act as secretary and writing down the child's account can help the younger, more reserved or intimidated child to voice an account of themselves.

Moving beyond the concrete

Neil, at 15 years of age, readily employed a host of psychological constructs in his self description or characterisation. When engaging young children, in particular, in exercises to elicit constructs, they may struggle to move beyond concrete, physical descriptions (such as their clothes, colour of hair, where they go to school and so forth) and not produce the psychological constructs which older children typically employ in elaborating their sense of identity.

Inviting the younger child to ladder a physical description may evoke meaningful psychological constructs. Thus asking a child if and why an elicited physical construct is important might proceed as follows:

Enquirer: 'Is it important that some children have freckles?'
Child: 'Yea.'
Enquirer: 'How come it's important?'
Child: 'Well kids with freckles are always telling jokes.'

There is generally a way to enable any young person to convey to the concerned enquirer a few of the key ways in which they understand themselves. Since it is highly unlikely that individuals develop one system for making sense of other people and an entirely separate system for making sense of themselves, a fruitful line of enquiry into self construing might start with an open-ended invitation such as: 'Tell me something about the other kids in your class'; 'What's this sister of yours like?'; or, 'So you have a pet dog called Rascal – tell me about him.'

Self portraits

Children who enjoy words often participate eagerly in the playful interrogations described above. Others prefer to express themselves visually, and find it easier to show or draw their image of themselves. The drawing in *Fig. 3.1* is by a 9-year-old boy whose mother saw him as something of an invalid because of an inherited calcium deficiency. The impression his self portrait gave was of a robust, active youth, a

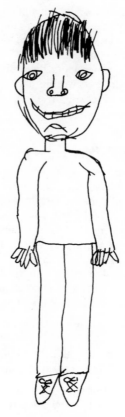

Fig. 3.1

view confirmed by his commentary on the picture: 'I'm one of the strongest boys in my class. Nobody pushes me around.'

Sometimes simple stylised portrayals of faces with a variety of facial expressions can open up fruitful conversations with children. Presenting a sketch of a child's face looking angry can encourage a child to describe his own feelings. The enquirer might ask:

- 'How do you guess this person's feelings?'
- 'Do you ever feel like that?'
- 'What thoughts go through your mind when you feel that way?'

Where children show an inclination to draw, Ravenette has suggested that they might be invited to sketch their feelings as in a 'portrait gallery'. *Fig. 3.2* shows the portrait gallery of a 9-year-old boy, Tom,

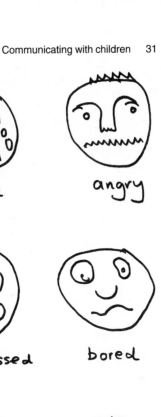
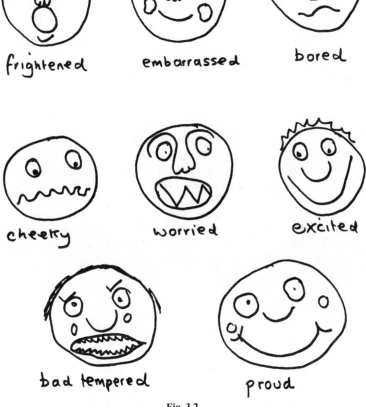

happy   sad   angry

frightened   embarrassed   bored

cheeky   worried   excited

bad tempered   proud

Fig. 3.2

who was struggling emotionally to cope with a foster placement with foster parents who were undertaking this care for the first time.

Tom was asked firstly to draw a happy face. He was then asked about times that made him feel happy. This was followed up by an inquiry as to whether Tom knew any other feelings and, as before, he was asked to draw the face and comment on his own experiences of the feeling. Tom came up with eleven faces. His responses to each were as follows:

- Happy – 'When I do things right.'
- Sad – 'When I fight with my big brother and get told off.'
- Angry – 'When people call me names; when I argue with my brother; when I shout at mum.'
- Frightened – 'Never feel frightened.'
- Embarrassed – 'Never.'
- Bored – 'At school when I've finished work; on holiday when I've nothing to do.'
- Cheeky – 'When I argue with mum.'
- Worried – 'About being fostered.'
- Excited – 'When I win things; when I'm going on trips and to the caravan.'
- Bad tempered – 'When I get sent to bed.'
- Proud – 'When I'm good at school; when I get an award.'

Providing a context

Drawings may also provide an effective stimulus to enable children to give a more detailed account of their construing in particular settings. Tom Ravenette (1977) pioneered the use of artfully vague cartoons that convincingly set a scene without making explicit exactly what's going on between the characters portrayed. His 'Trouble in school' caricatures offer the young person a range of educational scenarios from which to select three particularly appealing pictures; the example in *Fig. 3.3* is one of Ravenette's sketches. A child may be engaged in conversation with the enquirer along the following lines:

- 'Someone in this picture is feeling troubled. Which character do you think it is?'
- 'What do you think is happening?'
- 'What do you imagine they are thinking?'
- 'Why are they feeling this way?'
- 'What do you guess would make a difference to the way this person feels?'

With a little invention, this notion of sketching in a background on which the young person can impose a more personal sense, can focus

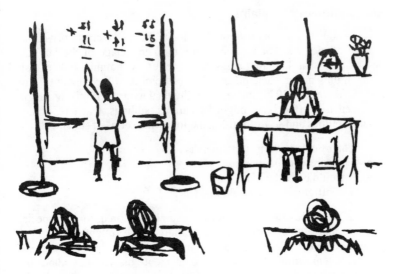

Fig. 3.3

discussions on other situations with particular importance for individual children. For example the scene in *Fig. 3.4* is from a series of illustrations unoriginally entitled 'Hurt in hospital' developed to encourage children with chronic illnesses to articulate what they make of their various medical encounters.

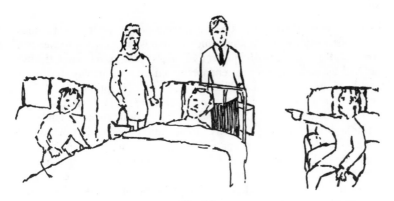

Fig. 3.4

Elaboration of complaints

It is, of course, possible to provide a focus for a conversation without
the use of pictures. For instance Kelly took advantage of the familiar
observation that human beings seem to enjoy nothing better than
complaining about each other. The 'elaboration of complaints' approach (Ravenette 1977) invites the individual to air their misgivings on
a chosen issue (the issue might be parents, siblings, teachers, grand-
parents, bullies and so forth) using the following series of statements:

- 'The trouble with most brothers is ...'
- 'They are like that because ...'
- 'It would be better if ...'
- 'The difference that would make is ...'

Such a sentence-completion format can be tailored to the special
interests and problems of particular children. The following extract is
from a personally designed questionnaire completed by a 10-year-old
boy with leukaemia who seemed to 'act out' his feelings about his
illness but could give no explanation to his mother as to why he
behaved as he did:

- 'What Leeds United needs is ... *a new good player.*'
- 'The worst thing about having cancer is ... *getting my needle put in my portacath.*'
- 'My mum ... *always does the washing.*'
- 'I wish ... *I did not have cancer.*'
- 'I get angry when ... *my needle gets put in my portacath.*'
- 'The best thing about school is ... *I like doing art.*'

Story-telling

There are evident similarities between the way Ravenette uses pictures
to provide the structure around which a youngster is invited to weave a
story, and the range of 'projective' tests that psychoanalytically-
inclined psychologists use to encourage children to display the 'inner
world' of their experience. The Children's Apperception Test (CAT),
for example, uses cartoon drawings of various animals (lions, monkeys,
dogs, even kangaroos) which are depicted in various scenes intended to
promote discussion of potentially problematic issues within the family
(such as sibling rivalry, or parental conflict). The user of the CAT
expects the child's accounts of what's going on in the picture to reflect
what's going on inside the child. The material produced is then
analysed within the psychologist's framework of Freudian child development theory.

The personal construct approach to the analysis of children's stories is significantly different. Certainly a personal construct psychologist designs what they hope will be personally salient cues to enable a young person to tell their particular tale. They may use pictures to establish a context, or provide prompts to maintain the momentum of a spoken account. However, there is no assumption that the experience of any character described in the story parallels precisely the experience of the story-teller. Rather the expectation is that, in telling their tale, the child will employ constructs that they use in their understanding of other people.

There is, further, an expectation that the range of ideas a child has evolved to try and make sense of those around them is also likely to form the foundations of a developing theory of self. It is nonetheless awfully tempting to check out with some children whether their responses to a story-telling exercise are, in fact, a thinly-veiled auto-biographical account of their own experiences. We might therefore suggest to a child that, 'We're really talking about you here, aren't we, Katie?' Such smart alec attempts at confirming the adult's hypotheses can sadly bring an enjoyable experiment to an abrupt and clumsy conclusion. An alternative way of pursuing the same hunch might be to ask:

- 'Are there any ways in which you think you are similar to the girl in the story Katie?', and
- 'What about the ways in which you think you and the girl are different from each other?'

Such wording emphasises more of an interest in the child's theories about human nature, rather than the psychologist's theories about children! In trying to create a psychological model that reflects the complex ways in which a young person's views 'fit together', there is a search to explore the intricacy of the *child's* construct system, rather than slot the child conveniently into any of the *enquirer's* predetermined diagnostic categories.

Organisation of construct systems

Once a young person has been able to articulate some of the ways in which they make sense of their world, there may be a wish to consider which discriminations matter most to the individual. Kelly proposed that individuals organise their constructs in a loosely hierarchical fashion with a limited number of what he dubbed 'core constructs' that are of central importance to our comprehension of events. One of Kelly's last PhD students, Dennis Hinkle, developed a number of neat ways of investigating these ordinal relationships between constructs. Hinkle (1965) devised a method of questioning, which he termed 'laddering', that rapidly leads to the heart of a person's belief system; 'why?' and 'how come?' questions are useful in this respect. Returning to Neil's self characterisation (described earlier in this chapter), questions which might lead towards his core constructs are:

- 'How come it is better to be tough than vulnerable?'
- 'Why do you believe it's important to be able to communicate your ideas?'
- 'What are the disadvantages of finding it difficult to make friends?'

At other times the enquirer might find he needs more detail to grasp the meaning of certain statements in a self characterisation. Hinkle developed an alternative style of questioning, which he called 'pyramiding', for checking out what a construct implies in practice. This relies on 'what?' and 'how?' questions. Ways of developing a better understanding of what Neil means by particular expressions in his self characterisation might include:

- 'Give me an example of a time when you felt you made a fool of yourself.'
- 'What sort of person do you think makes mistakes when talking in a large group?'
- 'How would I know you'd said something stupid?'

Resistance to change

One indication of superordinary, in Kelly's parlance, of one construct over another is if the individual considers that changing their view of themselves in one respect (e.g. becoming less popular at school) would automatically result in their revising their opinion of themselves in some other way (e.g. feeling less confident). These interrelationships can be mapped using an implications grid (another of Hinkle's ideas) but a simple clinical example serves to illustrate the principle:

> Brian, at 17 years old, had a chronic problem of encopresis. His soiling was a source of friction in his relationship with his mother. Moreover he had few friends and was more dependent on his family than most boys his age.
>
> He was offered admission to a residential treatment unit for adolescents. Staff in the unit were undecided about whether to focus the treatment regime on encouraging Brian to become more age-appropriately autonomous, or to concentrate on relieving his 'symptomatic' problem of soiling.

When Brian was consulted he was able to clarify the relationship between these two issues in his own mind. If he became more independent that would be fine but it would not, in his judgement, have any necessary influence on how likely he was to continue soiling. If however he were to become clean Brian reckoned there would be a veritable domino effect on other ways in which he construed himself, such as feeling more grown up, more attractive to girls, and more independent of his family.

The unit took Brian's opinion seriously and organised a treatment programme designed to tackle his soiling problem directly. As Brian had predicted, movement on this symptomatic construct set up a virtuous circle and boosted his self esteem no end.

This positive outcome illustrates how shifting position on a super-ordinate construct has a substantial knock-on effect on the rest of the system. Because such movement has so many implications, revisions of core construing can also prove to be the most resistant to change.

Grids

Personal construct theory is strongly associated with the use of the repertory grid technique devised by Kelly as a mathematical means of defining the relationship between elements and constructs. A number of more or less straightforward statistical packages are available to analyse significant patterns in a person's responses to these grid investigations: do certain elements cluster together?; are a particular pair of constructs used in a similar fashion?; and so forth. Computing power multiplies exponentially the number of calculations that can be made on the basis of a quite limited data set.

However the purpose of inquiry is to listen closely to what young people have to say. There is a danger that the unwary might be fooled into thinking that the messy business of understanding children can be subcontracted to a computer software program. It is however possible to use the inventive structure of repertory grids without needing an advanced degree in mathematics. Again a case illustration makes the point:

Jack (6) and Jill (7) are brother and sister who have lived in a series of foster homes since being admitted into the care of their local authority social services department as a result of concerns that they had been neglected by their own parents. Long-term decisions were now to be made about their future care arrangements. Their father (now remarried) had applied to have his children returned to live with him; Jack and Jill's current foster parents wished to make a long-term commitment to their care; social services' preference was to place the children with adoptive parents. The Children Act, under which their case was to be heard, demands that wherever possible the children whose wellbeing is under consideration be given a voice in proceedings.

Both Jack and Jill completed a very simple repertory grid. The elements they were asked to think about were the five homes they could remember living in. These were:

Mum and her partner
Dad and his new wife
Ron and Mary – first pair of foster parents (emergency reception)
Nick and Carol – second pair of foster parents (short-term allocation)
Andy and Ann – current foster parents (for more than a year).

Neither Jack nor Jill could recall the time when they lived with both their natural parents.

The names of each couple were written on postcards and Jack and Jill added small drawings to remind themselves of who was whom. They then completed a ranking grid by placing the elements (the five homes) in order of preference regarding the following questions:

- 'Who did you feel most safe with?'
- 'And who did you feel next most safe with?', and so on.

Jack and Jill undertook this task separately. The patterns of their replies were internally consistent, and they also showed a broad consensus in their preferences. The structure of the repertory grid allowed them to express their views on their future care in a way that the Court could both trust and respect.

Further discussion of the design, application, analysis and interpretation of various forms of grid are found in Fransella and Bannister (1977).

Dependency grids

Kelly devised one further specialised grid which can prove particularly pertinent to understanding children. The 'situational resources' grid maps the problems that confront a person against the sources of help that they can call upon for assistance. The theoretical underpinning of this matrix is Kelly's assertion that we are all dependent; what matters is how we disperse our dependencies. A healthy situational resources grid will indicate a range of people to whom a young person might turn for help and a strategic sense of which person is best equipped to help with a particular sort of difficulty. So a teenage daughter might happily seek her father's advice on possible career options, but would infrequently canvas his opinion on her choice of make-up!

Research into the intriguing phenomenon of 'resilient' children who manage to survive potentially damaging experiences of deprivation or disadvantage without suffering long-term harm to their psychological development has pointed to the importance of social support systems as a primary protective factor promoting the capacity to cope under duress. 'Born survivors' seem to make good use of extrafamilial supports and show an ability to recruit concerned allies to their cause. Conversely, children who keep all their emotional eggs in one basket and exhibit an undispersed pattern of dependency may struggle to cope when confronted with problems, if their sole source of support is either unavailable or ill-suited to provide some specialist form of help. School-phobic children sometimes find themselves in precisely such a dilemma.

The following case example illustrates how well a dependency grid can display the pattern of a young person's reliances on others. Peter, age 12, had had a urostomy as an infant and so is required to use a urine bag which needs fairly careful management. His family and physician considered he was of an age when it would be appropriate for him to take more responsibility for his own health care. As the dependency grid in *Table 3.1* shows, Peter felt far from prepared for such a promotion. Also of interest is that his willingness to delegate responsibilities was not restricted to issues surrounding 'the bag'. For example he does not see either doing his homework or cleaning his teeth as exclusively or even primarily his job.

Table 3.1 Peter's dependency grid

Whose job is it?

0 Not their job at all				7 Completely their job	

Task	Me	Mum	Dad	Sister	Gran	Friend
Cleaning teeth	4	5	6	0	0	0
Tidying my room	2	6	5	3	0	0
Taking my tablets	4	5	0	0	4	0
Buying and choosing my clothes	4	5	3	0	0	0
Spending money on me	3	4	0	0	3	0
Checking 'the bag'	4	5	2	0	1	0
Changing 'the bag'	4	7	0	0	3	0
Doing my homework	4	0	5	2	0	0

Conclusion

Personal construct theory does not provide a recipe book of techniques to guide us in designing our interventions in the lives of children. Kelly reckoned that the question 'why?' needed to be answered before the question 'how?' could be properly considered. This principled position can prove damnably frustrating for the hard-pressed practitioner wanting to know what to do next. This chapter has introduced readers into a range of ways in which they might tap the 'inside story' of a young person's experience. The remaining chapters will hopefully provide some insight into how this approach can be employed in putting this hard-won understanding to practical use.

Chapter 4

The exploration of self

'I'd rather exercise my mind than physical skill and strength'

Bear in mind Harry's age. He was 8 years old when he first entered the clinic, somewhat shy and naturally hesitant. He had been referred by his general practitioner because of poor concentration at school and 'general behaviour out of character for him', which by implication seemed to suggest behaviour which was causing a concern to others. Harry's reticence evaporated fairly rapidly over the first few sessions as he began to describe his predicament and the struggle to be understood.

It seemed important to develop an understanding of his 'character', and equally to discern the perceived change in character. Kelly's proposition that behaviour can be viewed as an experiment suggested that maybe Harry was trying out something new. Perhaps he was being aggressive in the Kellyan sense of actively elaborating some aspect of himself. That others were construing Harry's change of behaviour with concern did not necessarily imply that Harry perceived it in this way.

As Harry's story unfolded he demonstrated remarkable and astute observations of himself. His powers of self analysis appeared all but fully fledged. Reflection is an interpretative act, a means whereby we construe the way we are. As Bannister (1983) suggested, our failures to anticipate some of our own actions or make sense of them retrospectively assures us that self, like the world at large, is a mixture of the known and the mysterious. Perhaps it is the Piagetian influence that leads us to consider children as acting with self interest rather than with self knowledge. Perhaps this is also why Harry's self reflecting nature comes as a surprise. However the capacity to reflect upon our thoughts and actions is a defining characteristic of self, as understood in personal construct theory. As Bannister (1983) again illuminated reflexivity is the ability to distinguish the self that screams from the self that ponders why it screamed. Harry had grasped this. It seemed he had fathomed the meaning of much of his behaviour, and yet despite his ponderings much remained a mystery.

Background

Harry's family had something of a complicated history. His father never married his mother. His mother had subsequently married another man, had another son, and divorced him. Harry's father, for the last 3 years, was again, somewhat turbulently, living within the family. Harry suffered with occasional bouts of migraine and asthma, but nothing else medically of note.

At school Harry was described as very quiet, preferring his own company, his concentration likely to wander especially when required to listen, and showing a vulnerability to 'distraction by other classroom activities or things outside the classroom which catch his eye'.

An assessment of cognitive functioning illustrated both Harry's high level of ability across a broad spectrum of intellectual activity and literacy and also, in marked contrast, his unease with visuomotor tasks and consequent struggle to master mathematical concepts. It does appear that the two often go hand in hand. A difficulty in assimilating visuospatial information seems inextricably to hinder a child's command of mathematics. A dilemma for Harry, and children like him, was not the issue of being dim at maths – indeed many children come to such a conclusion relatively easily, and sometimes with relief – but that his inability in this one area stood out in stark contrast to his assessment of himself in pretty much all other academic areas. Indeed Harry would experience much validational support for his notion of himself as bright, but would have found himself at sea in terms of validation when it came to maths.

Experience of self *versus* the observation of self

Harry might therefore have been considered not only a source of perplexity for others, but also something of a mystery to himself. Sharon Jackson and Don Bannister (1985) carefully elaborated the idea that many children may appear confusing to other people (in that it seems difficult to understand them) but are perfectly able to derive an understanding of themselves. So where parents might feel like pulling their hair out in being unable to fathom why a child won't stop fighting his siblings, the child himself may knowingly take this stance out of choice. The child's fighting endorses his particular view of self.

The flipside of Jackson and Bannister's thesis is that other children can be both confusing to others and confusing to themselves. A catalogue of confusing experiences (such as Harry's mathematical ability, his illness, his father's return, the change in parental reactions to him, his social isolation and so forth) could invalidate a child's self construing to such an extent that the child becomes both a mystified and mystifying psychologist.

Self construing

Harry's construing of self became a central question. However the notion of self is something of a theoretical and conceptual minefield. Definitions of self abound. Many are esoteric and the interchangeability of terminology is perhaps unsurpassed in psychological literature. Notions such as self image, self concept, self worth and self esteem are customarily used synonymously.

Personal construct theory postulates that the notion of self is an act of construing like any other. We make sense of ourselves in the same manner that we make sense of other events. As other people play such significant roles in an individual's life, the ways in which we elaborate our construing of self must therefore be essentially similar to those ways in which we elaborate our construing of others. Self construing is an integral part of our total construct system. Whether we contrast or align ourselves with others we inevitably accept that 'without' and 'within' are perceived in the same terms. Thus we construe ourselves on constructs we also employ to construe others. As Bannister (1983) portrayed, our 'self picture and world picture are painted on the same canvas and with the same pigments'.

The self picture metaphor implies further that the self is also the artist. The active search for similarity ('that's just like me') and contrast ('you'd never see me like that') generates a sense of differentiation in self awareness. As the individuality corollary states, people differ from others in the way they construe events, and also therefore in the way they construe themselves. Such views led Bannister (1983) to define self as *not* a haphazard collection of autobiographical data, but what you believe yourself to be.

This context sharpens up a working model of self image as a non-evaluative description of what you perceive yourself to be: the identification of yourself along dimensions or constructs important to you. This contrasts with self esteem, which, being an evaluative aspect of self, can be viewed as the person's estimate of self (where they are) against where they would like to be.

Self image profile

In a search to find a way of representing a child's vision of self and leaning on the maxims of personal construct theory, Butler (1994) developed the Self Image Profile. *Table 4.1* shows one completed by Harry.

The profile has a set of self descriptions down the left hand side, along which children are invited to rate where they estimate they consider themselves to be. Only one pole of the construct is shown which facilitates the child in making ratings. Children as young as 6

Table 4.1 A Self Image Profile completed by Harry

Name   HARRY

Complete the self image scale by shading or ticking the most relevant box.

Item no.	How would you describe yourself?	Not at all 0	1	2	3	4	5	Very much so 6
1	Kind					▨●		
2	Friendly					▨●		
3	Confident			▨		●		
4	Happy			▨				●
5	Lively				▨		●	
6	Helpful				▨		●	
7	Honest						▨●	
8	Tidy				▨		●	
9	Feel different from others							▨●
10	Lazy	●			▨			
11	Lonely		●			▨		
12	Stubborn							▨●
13	Moody			●	▨			
14	Worrier				▨●			
15	Nervous		●	▨				
16	Shy			●	▨			
17	Easily upset		●			▨		
18	Frightened	●	▨					
19	Bad tempered			●		▨		
20	Angry				●	▨		

▨ 'as I am'; ● 'as I'd like to be'.

years, with the assistance of an adult to read out the descriptions, are able to complete the profile.

The self image profile is designed around principles central to personal construct theory in determining the clinical utility of any test or psychometric instrument (Winter 1992). Firstly, items are of necessity, meaningful to the population for whom the scale is designed, and are representative of events in the child's life. Thus the self descriptions, or constructs, are child generated and therefore of familiar and relevant parlance.

For the Self Image Profile the self descriptions were generated from a wide sample of children invited to comment on themselves in the customary format of construct elicitation. Thus the sample were asked to compare and contrast themselves with other people so that a wide variety of constructs were generated. From this large sample of elicited descriptions of self, themes which commonly emerged were selected as the self descriptions for the profile.

Secondly the profile regards the 'raw data' – the information provided by the child – as of paramount importance. There is no attempt to convert the child's responses to fit the theoretical or mathematical constructs of those who administer the questionnaire.

Thirdly, flexibility is built in. The self descriptions are not 'written in stone' as descriptions can be altered or removed and new constructs drafted in to meet the needs of the situation. An example of a modified version is illustrated in Chapter 7 (*Table 7.3*). The flexible nature of the Self Image Profile is one of its assets. The crux of any scale is that it reflects what is important to the person filling it in.

What of validity, a concept embraced so lovingly by psychologists? Validity, in both its content and construct forms, respectively seeks to inquire as to the scale's potency in measuring a representative sample of the behaviour domain to be measured and to the scale's ability to test the theoretical trait under investigation. Given the child-generated nature of the self descriptions in the Self Image Profile, seeking validity measures seems nothing short of superfluous. Kelly (1955) equated validity with usefulness and increased understanding. If the profile makes sense to the child, taps his vision of self and reveals patterns that the therapist can usefully harness, then it will have served its purpose.

Children are invited to rate themselves, using a Likert scale, anchored with 0 (not at all) and 6 (very much so). Harry made two ratings – the first concerning how he felt about himself at the present time, and the second citing how he would wish to be (his ideal). These are illustrated in *Table 4.1*. Many different aspects of self can of course be evaluated by inviting the child to rate for example, 'as I used to be'; 'as I'm expected to be'; 'as I was before the accident' and so forth.

Harry's first rating – how I am – might be taken to represent his self image. His ratings along the constructs represent what Bannister (1983) alluded to as the self picture. The visual display of the profile immediately depicts how a child construes himself. This is shared knowledge. It demands no complicated scoring strategy or correlational analysis which has a tendency to quash the child's original response. Further, there is no lie scale, a brainchild of the suspicious. The Self Image Profile accepts, in contrast, the child's statements about self credulously. It acknowledges the child's 'raw' scores as illustrative of his sense of self.

For the computational, the Self Image Profile can be scored. Butler (1994) suggested that items 1–7 portray the desired end of self statements, so that a cumulative high score on these 7 items gives an indication of positive self regard. Harry's score was 22 which is suggestive of a patchy and wanting positive self image. In contrast, items 10–20 depict the more undesirable pole of self statements, so summing these scores provides a measure of the child's negative sense of self. Harry's score of 38 is relatively high and suggests he construed himself in quite a negative light.

Properties of the Self Image Profile

The Self Image Profile has been found to correlate significantly with the Coopersmith self esteem scale, although it has been argued that the two scales measure different aspects of self (Butler *et al.* in preparation). The Coopersmith is unidimensional with a question format implying evaluative judgements, and might therefore be considered to tap the child's self esteem.

In contrast the Self Image Profile, with the items generated by children, seeks to gather the child's portrayal of self in a non-judgemental way. It might therefore be considered to tap the child's self image. However, as described later, inviting the child to make a second rating of self – in terms of 'how I would like to be' – can lead to an understanding of the child's self esteem. The discrepancy between the ratings 'how I am' and 'how I would like to be' is such a measure. Factor analysis of the Self Image Profile has produced 6 robust factors which appear to separate the positive and negative descriptions. In terms of psychometric properties the Self Image Profile therefore appears a valid instrument.

However the attraction of the profile perhaps lies not so much in its mathematical properties, but in its root assumptions which stress the importance of items being generated by the population for which it is designed for – children in this case – not by the experimenter who wishes to observe the population. In Winter's terminology, the Self

Image Profile concerns itself with the client's, not the clinician's yard-stick (Winter 1992). By adopting such a stance, items assume greater meaning.

Self esteem

There is a fancy within personal construct theory that self esteem, being an evaluative aspect of self, is characterised by the individual's perceived distance between where they are and where they would ideally wish to be.

Thus a person who perceives of their ideal as achievable and within reach might be considered to have a reasonably high self esteem whereas someone who senses a wide gulf between perceived self and how they would like to be might be considered to be experiencing low self esteem. Interestingly it might be argued that where a person considers there is very little, if any, discrepancy between self and idealised self, they might experience a sense of complacency.

A second rating of 'how I'd like to be' on the Self Image Profile enables the distance between self and ideal to be observed and calculated. Harry's self esteem, therefore, could be calculated by observing the size of the discrepancy between self and ideal on all items and summing the discrepancies. In Harry's case his self esteem score would therefore be 30. Harry's profile illustrates a fairly consistent discrepancy, although he also indicates no wish for change in terms of kindness, friendliness, honesty, feeling different from others, stubbornness and being a worrier. The profile highlights where Harry wishes to change. In particular he would prefer to be happier and more confident, less lazy, lonely or as easily upset. A therapeutic agenda is therefore apparent. Employing the Self Image Profile as a directional aid to therapy is discussed in Chapter 6.

Such notions suggest that change in self construing is a therapeutic aim. However Bannister and Agnew (1977) have argued that permanence is a central characteristic of self. They assert that self is constructed and elaborated over time, which might be construed as an act of self creation, and yet our core constructs maintain the person as a person. It is as if, although we recognise fluctuation, shifts and transformations in the way we construe ourselves over time, the essential 'me-ness' remains the same.

A further characteristic of self, according to Bannister and Agnew (1977) is our separateness. We each entertain a notion of our own separateness from others, and it is this separateness which enables us to formulate contrasts between ourselves and others.

In a later, unpublished work Bannister (1983) elaborated his notions of self, inviting the consideration of a superordinate structure or series of 'professional' constructs as a means of understanding self. Harry will be considered in relation to these means of construing.

Notion of individuality

This rotates around whether a person perceives an individual stance as legitimate. As a construct it might be phrased as an awareness and acknowledgement of self as an individual with a willingness to discuss and explore one's individuality *versus* a stance where individuality is perceived as self indulgent, egotistical, narcissistic or big-headed.

How an individual aligns himself along such a construct is inevitably culturally determined. Thus western values tend to emphasise the importance of the individual compared to other cultures where the whole is perceived as more important than the individual. Other experiences which favour collective rather than individualistic construing might include entering the armed forces or religious sects where commonality of construing is paramount. Ironing out individuality is a stated aim.

In the realm of the young, Piagetian opinion of egotistical development in early childhood suggests children (at least, western children) are naturally engaged in elaborating the 'I'. In more advanced years adolescence is oft characterised by a feverish and impatient search for independence and individuality. Both are traditionally construed as necessary and healthy by society even though they seem inevitably to stretch parental composure, patience and tolerance, sometimes to the extreme.

Children search for both individuality and commonality of construing. Distinctiveness is apparent in the child's ubiquitous sense that things are never fair with the child's wish for his or her needs to be recognised by others, despite parents testifying that they treat everyone 'equally and alike'. On the other hand children also search to present a picture of unity and commonality, such as is apparent in allegiances to sport teams, social groups and current fashions.

There was an emphatic sense that Harry construed himself as an individual. He dressed 'old fashionably' and as *Table 4.1* illustrates, he not only had a feeling that he was different from others but he had no wish to change that. Harry valued his separateness from others. He preferred being on his own or being in adult company rather than mixing with other children. As he said, 'I don't like the company of other children'. Harry intimated that the origin of his sense of difference was because he considered he had an 'adult mind'. He enlarged on this by figuring he was able to find solutions to problems independently. For example he expressed concern over his mum and dad arguing but kept it in check by 'taking the right precautions' and 'making decisions so I don't worry'.

A further illustration of Harry's sense of uniqueness was apparent in his perception of himself as stubborn, again an aspect of himself he had no desire to change. According to Harry, when he decided to make something happen he stuck to doing what he felt was right rather than be moulded, undermined or influenced by other people's points of view.

Notion of a sense of history

The contrast Bannister (1983) elaborated here was between employing one's biography as a thread, a narrative elaborated over a time line therefore enabling the individual to link vividly the past to present self, *versus* the sense of living more or less in the here and now so the image of self, to quote Bannister, 'elides the past into a limited catalogue of events which are seen dimly and as of little present relevance'.

The stories individuals have regarding their development rarely fit the developmental stages outlined in texts on child development. Phil Salmon (1970) has discussed this idea fully. More usually children reflect on their own development by noting 'watershed points'. Perhaps events perceived as trivial to others may have an enormously significant and lasting influence in creating a notion of self. For Harry, there might be a tendency to look towards the trauma of family changes as being influential in his development. Life event theory and much behavioural analysis might anticipate such an occurrence to have had a significant effect on moulding his view of self. However personal construct theory accords the individual's construing of an event, not the event itself, with greater importance. What was significant to Harry might well prove to be something not necessarily anticipated by an interested 'other'.

The experience corollary, which states that a person's construction system varies as they successively construe the replication of events, might help to further this point. We change our view of self in relation to the accuracy of our anticipations. Thus we might, as a child, perceive ourselves to be mature, self assured and reasonably streetwise, until perhaps innocently but disparagingly another child on a school trip points out how neatly our lunch box is packed. Suddenly the child's constructions about self, regarding maturity and independence are found wanting. Kellyan hostility might help preserve the child's sense of maturity – he may resort to bullying and taunting the child who made the comment in order to reduce the potency of the remark. Alternatively, the child in accounting for how he has acquired such a well presented lunch with all its trimmings, might make a revision in self construing and begin to entertain the notion that he really is something of a 'mummy's boy'. Thus 'trivial' events can have prodigious personal significance.

Harry appeared to possess a clear sense of personal history. He considered himself as intelligent, bright, perfectionist and never satisfied, confident but not overconfident. He ventured the idea that others tend to become overconfident 'because they are not bothered about how good they are'. However Harry also acknowledged a tendency to daydream and become distracted. He postulated that his mind 'plays tricks on me'.

Harry described that when he was about 7 he used to think the house was haunted with dead cats in the garden and dark pictures on the wall of people who used to live in the house. He lay awake at night, in fear, unable to sleep. With the resulting tiredness he found the next day's schoolwork perplexingly difficult and found himself drifting in and out of daydreams.

Such an experience clashed with his view of self as bright, particularly when his family and teacher would raise the issue of his daydreaming and distractibility. He reconstrued self as 'stupid', perhaps temporarily, and consequently suffered what Kelly (1955) called 'slot rattling' along the construct bright *versus* stupid. Harry was switching his view of self between the contrasting poles, on some occasions perceiving himself as bright and at other times as stupid. This is an unsettling change. Given that intelligence was a core construct for Harry, and the wide ranging implications possibly experienced with a reconstruction of himself as stupid, he may have experienced threat – an awareness of comprehensive change in one's core (self) structures. A possible solution when core constructions of self are under threat, and one considered by Harry, is the contemplation of suicide.

Notion of personal change

Bannister (1983) suggested here the contrast between the idea that our basic character remains the same throughout our life *versus* a viewpoint which stresses development, choice and elaboration. The perception of self as unchanging is deterministic and often genetically loaded. It generates statements such as 'I am not one for socialising', 'I'm just like my dad in his love of music', 'I was brought up to respect other people's property'. Such a view contrasts with that which recognises the personal responsibility for change in the evolution of self. Examples here might include 'I used to dread public speaking but now I find it exhilarating' and 'I'm going to bring up my child very differently from how I was brought up'.

Harry appeared to favour the view of self as stuck. For example Harry had only one friend. He said, 'I'm not one for going around making friends. I'd rather be alone'. As for sporting endeavours Harry showed an even greater aversion. 'I'd rather exercise my mind than physical skill and strength', was how he responded to a question about his liking for sport. Further, Harry had erected a stance concerning his behaviour which seemed an unlikely bet for change. He remarked, 'I keep out of trouble. I keep quiet. In that way I don't get noticed'. Finally his view of his appearance seemed fixed and not amenable to change. He said, 'I don't look very nice. When it comes to it, it doesn't really matter'.

Notion of public self *versus* private self

Bannister (1983) argued that this issue revolves around the degree to which we choose to communicate our vision of ourselves *versus* the degree to which we conceal or seek to retain secrecy over our self. Some individuals openly express their views whilst others may be reserved over talking about themselves, protective over who knows what about them and only occasionally, if at all, let their 'guard down'.

Harry seemed to be struggling in both domains. His public self – intelligent, someone who reads a lot, able to talk with adults – succeeded in his relationships with adults but failed miserably in his attempts to get on with children. In his words he speculated that 'kids don't understand me'. Harry had therefore manufactured another public self for when he was with children, a major experiment in self creation, where aspects of self were generated anew. Harry told the tale: 'I've made a character up at school. Stupid. Dummy. I act like I'm stupid. Others understand me easier. I make jokes up. They think I'm stupid. At least they don't pick on me or beat me up. They leave me alone. Then I'm all right'.

Harry's experience seems to fit well with Miller Mair's (1977a) contention that we often construct our selves as 'fortresses set up against a hostile world and assume, on the psychological plane, that the Englishman's home is still his castle'. Harry was able, it seemed, to construe himself as both bright and stupid depending upon the context in which he was functioning at any one time. In formulating a protective public persona concerned with being stupid, Harry was in effect developing a 'splinter self'. He appeared easily to be able to step in and out of a new 'stupid' self at will.

Miller Mair (1977b) developed an idea around the self as a community. He postulated that individuals may adopt very different, often contrasting, roles in different contexts, each role with its own self history, anticipatory nature and validational history. The common phenomenon of a child behaving very differently at home from at school is a broad illustrative example. Of importance, in personal construct theory terms, is whether the child perceives of himself differently in these two contexts. Only if he does, might he be conceived as having two selves. Harry's description of himself as behaving as if he were in two minds – the private adult self and the dummy child self – is a lived experience of this notion of a community of selves.

The idea of the person living through different selves is not to regard the individual as pathological. It is an invitation to consider the individual as if they were able to take on different selves in making sense of the different and varied situations which confront them. Rather than being pathological, a community of selves may instead, enable the person to actively experience and explore the world from numerous perspectives. Having many vantage points from which to act might indeed enhance the individual's pursuit of making sense. To paraphrase Robert Bolt, could it be that Harry is 'a man for all seasons'.

Conclusion

Within personal construct theory the notion of self is considered to be an act of construing like any other event. An individual is best understood as making sense of himself through the same manner of construing that he employs in grappling with other events with which he is confronted. Thus if we are tempted to construe others along a dimension labelled 'stupid' *versus* the contrast 'bright', we are likely to align ourselves somewhere along just such a construct.

Eliciting a child's constructs therefore provides an opportunity to understand the dimensions they consider important both with respect to themselves and to others. Chapter 3 described a host of ways this might be accomplished. This chapter described a more formal means of accessing how children view themselves, utilising the Self Image Profile.

Kelly showed some hesitation about the manner in which formal assessments were designed and conducted. He was concerned that a test should address the following clinical issues, elaborated in Winter (1992):

- Does it reflect the construing of the client or the individual who devised the test? The Self Image Profile is composed of child-generated items, condensed into a manageable range of self descriptions according to a commonality of themes. As such the items increase the likelihood of being meaningful to the child. Kelly argued that given personal construct theory is primarily concerned with the viewpoint of its object of study – namely the child – any measures derived from the child are objective.

- Does it elicit permeable constructs, which enable an understanding of the here and now and an anticipation of the future, rather than being concerned purely with the individual's past? Items, particularly for young people, need to be alive and relevant. The need for flexibility – being able to modify and change according to the situation – compared to a rigid unforgiving framework, customarily apparent with many scales, is built into the Self Image Profile. The format of asking the child two question in relation to each self description – how you are now (present) and how you would wish to be (future) – seeks an understanding of both the child's predicament and idealised solution.

- Are the items representative of events in the child's life? By eliciting the items from a sample of children and locating the focus on aspects of self, their relevance and meaningfulness might be considered more appropriate than perhaps projective investigations where the child is faced with the challenge of construing the likes of ink blots.

- Do the items strike a balance between stability and sensitivity, being concerned both with areas the child perceives as constant or core, and dimensions or avenues along which the child wishes to change? The format of the Self Image Profile highlights those aspects where the child wishes to remain stable and those he regards as problematic. Further the child is able to estimate the degree to which he perceives a discrepancy between his notion of self and how he would wish to be. The profile thus reveals pathways along which the child wishes to move. In chapter 6, this notion is developed therapeutically.

- Is the outcome faithful to the data provided by the child? Unlike many other scales, the Self Image Profile has no hidden agenda; there is no intent to disguise the purpose of the scale; and there is no wish to catch the child out with lie scales. Further there is no over complicated scoring system, such as occurs with grid analysis which neglects the data provided by the child in favour of sophisticated correlational and cluster analyses.

- Does it reveal constructs which are communicable? By incorporating a visual profile the scale assures the child, in addition to interested others, of the result. The child can reveal, to himself and others, something about himself. The clinician or observer might then appreciate the child's perspective on himself and begin to acknowledge the importance of balancing the child's understanding of self with the customary emphasis upon the clinician's understanding of the child.

Chapter 5

Children struggling to achieve

'Look at me'

The ubiquitous cry of young children. In the playground, classroom, music lesson, sports field and swimming pool, children strive to achieve. Further they usually wish others to know about their successful deeds and exploits. 'Look what I've done' is not so much an appeal for attention but a request that the child's proficiency, mastery and competence are acknowledged.

Jacob Bronowski's (1973) compelling reflection that 'the most powerful drive in the ascent of man is the pleasure of his own skill. He loves to do what he does well and, having done it well, he loves to do it better' applies equally as well for children. Perhaps more so for children are energetically inclined to share the pleasures of their skills with others.

Validation of self

Jonathan Glover (1991) has argued that the need for recognition has at least three components. We wish others to see us at least roughly as we think we are. We want to be respected. And we want to be liked. Recognition of the way we would wish to be seen, by others who independently and freely give it, validates the view we have of ourselves.

Children eagerly seek confirmation of their skills, ability and efforts. However it may only prove meaningful to the child if it validates a notion he has about himself. A child who enjoys swimming for example will seek to have his own estimates of success validated. 'I did it! Did you see me? I swam without my armbands!' is a familiar shriek. Validation or recognition confirms a view of self. Children gladly accept a certificate or badge as further evidence of their competency.

Should, however, a child not be struck by the idea of being a swimmer but is presented to swimming classes to 'make' him a better swimmer, recognition of any success may conflict with his notions of self. Indeed he may seek to play the fool or stubbornly refuse to progress so that he does not have to face invalidation of his construing of self. Further, Susan Harter (1978) has argued that any 'external' rewards such as badges may reduce, not encourage, the child to engage further in the activity because it undermines the child's intrinsic desire to accomplish the goal. Either through avoidance of invalidation, or a sense that the child's intrinsic pleasure regarding achievement is falsified by overjustification, the child may drop the activity as soon as possible.

Competence, confidence and being a connoisseur

Competence might be described as the individual's estimate of their ability to undertake a task. Thus children might perceive themselves as good at certain tasks and perhaps simultaneously claim their incompetence in other areas. The appetite children have for what is construed to be within their capabilities with their claims of 'Watch me!' and 'Easy peasy!' contrasts markedly with a tendency to avoid undertakings they consider are beyond them.

Individuals might be regarded as connoisseurs of any endeavour, undertaking or activity over which they actively elaborate. Just as the artist is a dab hand with colour, perspective and contrast, the taxi driver has 'the knowledge' of street plans, the tennis player has an intricate understanding of the top spin lob, so too children might be considered expert in computer games, music, fashion or fishing. *Table 5.1* illustrates the depth of expertise one 10-year-old boy demonstrated in his judgement of football shirts.

Confidence might be conceptualised as related to the 'goodness of fit' between how an individual expects to perform and how they actually perform. There might be a sense of confidence (or lack of confidence) also in the person's anticipation of whether they will (or will not) meet their expectation. Thus a sense of confidence is anticipatory, whilst the feeling of confidence comes with how well the person's performance 'fits' with their expectation. Such a model of confidence adopts Mildred McCoy's (1977) notion of goodness of fit.

Where there is a discrepancy between expectation and performance, the person experiences guilt (they have behaved in a way they would not have anticipated of themselves). Such a model equally describes a person's lack of confidence in 'goodness of fit' terms as it does a person's sense of confidence.

Butler (1996) extended McCoy's notion of goodness of fit within the sporting context. This is illustrated in *Fig. 5.1*. What follows an estimate of efficacy or competence is crucial. Should the person's estimate be validated, there is goodness of fit. Thus when the

Table 5.1 A connoisseur of football shirts: the elaborated thoughts of a 10-year-old

Colour of the shirt
Different tones of colour
Whether a pattern was sewn into the shirt
Complicated or simple design
Stripes, hoops or full colour
Stripes, fuzzy or clear
Old-fashioned or modern design
Colour of trim
Elasticated trim
Texture of material

Sleeves different or same colour as shirt
Stripes down sleeve
Details on cuffs

Presence of collar
Colour of collar
Details on collar – striped or not
Buttons on collar or elasticated
Colour of buttons
Triangle on collar
Polo neck or 'v' shape

Whether sponsor's name is displayed
Type of sponsor [e.g. beer, computers]
Sponsor's colour
Whether sponsor's colour contrasts or blends with shirt colour
Sponsor's shape

Badge central or to the side
Shield around the badge
Badge size

Manufacturer's name displayed
Position of manufacturer's name [to the side or central]

competent piano player gives a virtuoso performance their expectation is confirmed and they experience confidence. A child who perceives themselves as good at maths experiences a goodness of fit and sense of confidence if they happen to do well in the maths test.

There is similarly a goodness of fit where a child's sense of ineptness is confirmed. A child's early attempts at perhaps learning to catch a ball is heralded with cries of 'It's too hard; I can't do it'. Their expectation seems well founded when a succession of catches fail to be held. The child's expectation is confirmed, leaving them reasonably confident that they are indeed pretty lousy at catching.

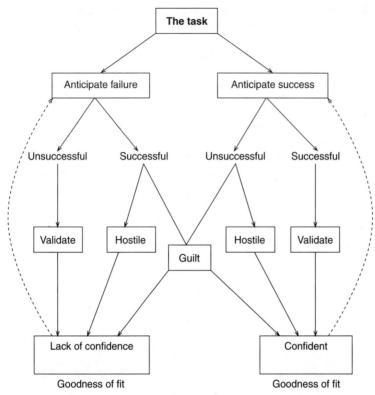

Fig. 5.1 A model of confidence, incorporating McCoy's 'goodness of fit' notion. Adapted from Butler (1996)

Intriguingly perfect performances are rare. Errors and mistakes creep into the performances of even the most adept and competent. In contrast, successes, perhaps infrequent, but successes nevertheless, emerge and litter the efforts of novice performers. When our predictions are temporarily or briefly invalidated there is a fleeting incongruity of goodness of fit and a flicker of hostility. Hostility in personal construct theory terms is the individual's effort to protect the view they have of themselves despite evidence to the contrary. They tamper with the evidence by rationalising, excusing or blaming. Hostility thus preserves the individual's sense of competence (or lack of confidence).

Thus the pianist who plays a wrong note or two maybe denies it, blames the conditions ('My hands were cold') or attributes it to tiredness. In contrast, a child who in endeavouring to catch the ball surprises him-

or herself by clutching feverishly to prevent the ball falling to the ground yells in amazement 'Did you see that?'. The tendency is to construe the success as if it were beginner's luck, thus again confirming the sense that ball catching is not as yet an expected or familiar experience and one the child cannot as yet feel confident about.

When an individual's estimate is consistently invalidated, guilt is experienced. Thus were the pianist to unremittingly hit the wrong notes, the experience might undermine the individual's view of self as competent. The consistent lack of a goodness of fit generates an acceptance that they are not perhaps as good as they thought, culminating in a loss of confidence. Yet again, conversely, a child's construction of self as incompetent in terms of ball catching will begin a reconstruing of self when his emerging skills bring him further success and enable him to predict his success. He too experiences guilt in accomplishing a task he imagined he was incapable of. Perhaps the child will then begin to revise the view of self from someone who can't catch balls to someone who is reasonably competent in such an activity.

Influence of others

Other people, engaged in a social role with the child, may undoubtedly play an influence in the child's estimate of competence. Children are the focus of much unprovoked and unsolicited advice as well as being recipients of needed support, inspiration and consolation. Parents, teachers, coaches and other children can seriously sway a child's sense of mastery.

There is fairly compelling evidence linking parental attributions and feelings towards a child with how the child construes him or herself (Rowe 1983; Butler *et al.* 1994). Parental annoyance, anger and intolerance towards a child in the guise of negative comments such as 'You're useless, give it here', places the child often in the position of internalising the feeling. Children hence blame themselves, indeed come to feel useless and maybe perceive themselves as not worthy.

At school, a child is potentially further at risk of construing himself as incompetent. Teachers who customarily focus their concerns and efforts on the child's ability and effort will inevitably at times evaluate the child as lacking in either ability or effort, or sometimes both. As far as gradings and test marks are perceived in comparative terms by the child there is an inherent vulnerability for a child to construe themselves as incompetent compared to others in class. A sense of not being any good is again potentially fostered.

The playing field, often the source of success and nourishment of competence may, for some, become a further arena in which incompetence is promoted. Error correction is indubitably a kernel of traditional coaching. A ceaseless focus on what a child is doing wrong generates the notion, and one often expressed, that 'I'm no good at that'. It is not surprising then that many children opt out of sporting, music and artistic endeavours at the earliest possible opportunity.

Peers may offer a safe haven. The compelling security of friendship may defuse much unwanted criticism and nurture the child's sense of competence. Those very acts of bravado and daring many children pursue in the company of other children may be seen as means of gaining credibility and 'currying favour' with their peers.

However, peers are also the source of much threat. Sometimes their actions undermine the child's notion of self as competent and raise the child's awareness, in a Kellyan sense, that sweeping changes in core construing may be imminent. The widespread taunts and jibes many children bear may focus the child's own attention on his incompetencies. The dread of social exclusion, by peers not allowing the child to join in shared activities, may leave a child feeling isolated, unusual and lacking in social competence. Flippant quips, jokes and banter along with more critical remarks about a child that he is no good, has to seek help, or has to have special needs, also endanger the child's notion of self as competent.

Coping by avoidance

Children of course cope with perceived incompetence in many ways. A child, for example, may opt out of activities such as sport, music, languages and art, thus avoiding further instances of incompetence, although the notion of self as incompetent is validated by the very experience of avoiding them. The commonplace and recurring affirmations we hear from adults as to their inability to play music or reflections about how bad they were at school with languages appears confirmation of their preparedness to construe themselves as incapable.

Interestingly Betty Edwards (1988) has discussed the joy many children experience in their early doodlings with pencil and paper and how they construct and share with delight their first drawings. She has eloquently argued that children who are then subsequently corrected in their art, as if there were a prescribed way of doing it, come to construe themselves as not good at it. They advance, both to themselves and to others, that they can't draw. Thus in middle childhood we see many children give up on drawing. They lay their frustrated and meddled experiences of drawing to rest. What they maintain is a sketchy but readily volunteered construction of themselves as pretty lousy in that department.

A continued struggle

Some areas of perceived incompetence, of course, cannot be so easily avoided. These have to be continually endured. Literacy, the agony of the unrecognised dyslexic, and numeracy are two such areas. A child's struggle with the experience of dyslexia is discussed in Chapter 7. As for the acquisition of mathematical concepts, Piaget interestingly, regarded the teacher's role as being intellectually non-interventionist and relatively unimportant; mathematics being essentially 'constructed by the children themselves'. The teacher who intervenes, he argued, may foster the child's sense of incompetence.

Margaret Donaldson (1984) predicted that children have considerable difficulty in learning mathematics whenever it is taught to them, because much of mathematics learnt in school is relatively 'disembedded' from the immediate context. Hughes (1986) has elaborated on this. He regards mathematics as a secret code, a code which contains a number of features which distinguish it from the informal mathematics children acquire before school. It is context free (what does two and two makes four refer to?) and rests heavily on written symbolism $(2 + 2 = 4)$.

Hughes argued that the difficulty for children in acquiring mathematical concepts lies in their difficulty in translating from one form of representation to another – from recognising that $6 - 2 = 4$ is a representation of 'me only having four sweets left if I give my sister two of them'. Written arithmetic problems serve no obvious purpose for the child first entering school. In order for it to be meaningful the child has to translate the problem into everyday usage. Hughes argued that the teacher's role might be best utilised in helping children translate – to see the advantages that grasping mathematical concepts might have for the child in his contact with the world. Hughes discussed how children who struggle with maths may not have been convinced that the journey of understanding is worth taking. The child needs help in deciding that the journey is indeed worth exploration. As Bannister and Fransella (1986) vividly surmised in relation to change, 'no one voluntarily walks the plank into the unknown depths of the ocean'. The teacher is of course pivotal in encouraging the child to walk the plank and take the plunge.

Fascinatingly, Kelly's initial thoughts when asked about how his theory applied to a child who failed to learn to read, were 'find out if the child likes the teacher!'*. It would indeed seem important to like one's mentor if you are to trust him to guide you through a venture so

---

*I am grateful to Tom Ravenette's comments here, as it was Tom who originally asked Kelly the question.

fraught with potential embarrassments and humiliations. A teacher's role from a construct theory perspective might best be conceptualised as one who encourages, with support, a child's tentative steps towards the unknown, always with vigilant recognition of his experiments and elaborations. Perhaps the most creative and inventive learning occurs when we aspire to teach in ways that a child learns best.

Susan Harter (1985) attempted to understand children's sense of competence through her scale, the self perception profile. It seeks the child's assessment of self in a variety of areas – social, appearance, sport, academic and behavioural. There is here an assumption that children who perceive of themselves as ineffective in such areas consider themselves to be incompetent. It may that they have a very elaborated notion of self at the contrast end. They may thus be connoisseurs of, as it were, incompetence.

Thus children who construe themselves as socially 'incompetent' may regard themselves as experts in aspects of social isolation. They construct well-validated notions of self as a loner and develop avenues of exploration based on this core understanding of self. The implications of being socially inept might include not being able to get along with others, finding other people's behaviour difficult to fathom, and whenever one tries to make a friend one gets rebuffed. When such experiences occur the child's construing of social self as incompetent is confirmed. The child opts to prefer his own company. He might go so far as to avoid all social contact, preferring to engage in the physical world, rather than the psychological world of people and having to comprehend the confusing rules that govern social behaviour.

Such extremes of social avoidance are seen with children who have Asperger's syndrome. Lorna Wing (1981) encapsulated the specific expertise such children often develop. They become intensely interested in one or two subjects such as steam trains, bus timetables, prehistoric monsters, fossils, to the exclusion of all else. They, as it were, become connoisseurs of asocial and idiosyncratic events. Being unable to anticipate the social reactions of others, such children seem unable to interact appropriately and may talk incessantly about something that holds their special interest despite other people's obvious boredom, or tend to make obscure, irrelevant or tactless remarks in company.

Nine-year-old Frances, referred for, amongst other problems, her very fussy eating, demonstrated her elaborate notions about food. Despite her avoidance of all but a few foods (fishcakes and cheese spread sandwiches being the notable exceptions), she was able to describe a reasonably elaborate set of constructs which she employed to evaluate any food she was faced with:

Crisp _____ Soft

Warm _____	Cold
Sweet _____	Not much taste
Don't need to be cooked _____	Food which is cooked
Smooth _____	Has bits/lumps in it
Gooey _____	Rock hard
Looks horrible _____	Looks yummy

The construct concerning consistency (smooth—has bits/lumps in it) seemed superordinate. Frances would not sample even the smallest morsel of food if she considered it to be lumpy. Food which was lumpy 'felt horrible' and made her 'feel sick'. Concentrating therefore on the smooth end of the construct Frances was invited to explore, and hopefully sample, food which she knew would not have lumps in. Apart from the sweet—not much taste dimension, Frances could determine the qualities of food along all her other constructs by merely looking at the food sample. Appearance influenced her choices greatly.

Interestingly Frances threw herself into this experiment and discovered that even food which looked horrible (baked potato), provided it was smooth, she was prepared to give it a try. Indeed she discovered she actually liked the taste of baked potato. Her very cautious sampling of smooth food led her to the discovery that whether food was crisp or soft, warm or cold, sweet or without much taste, cooked or not cooked, looking horrible or yummy, did not influence her sampling. Only rock hard food was avoided. Frances was then invited to consider both taste and smell in addition to appearance in her sampling of smooth and non-rock-hard food. She again tackled this with some enthusiasm and discovered a range of foods including seedless jam, cheese toasties, milk shakes and pancakes, which she actually liked.

Fay Fransella (1972) presented an in-depth discussion of how individuals who stutter become connoisseurs of that experience. They have elaborate notions of themselves as stutterers and little notion of what it would be like to be fluent. The implications of stuttering are known. In contrast, the implications of being fluent are ill understood. This explained why Fransella was able to help such individuals develop fluency, but they found it extremely difficult to be fluent. The final hurdle – seeing self as fluent – was the most difficult. They would demonstrate a high level of fluency but, as if loathe to leave the known self behind – that of stutterer – they would occasionally revert to stuttering.

The difficulty in changing is often embodied in a lack of understanding of what the change will imply. A change in behaviour might occur, perhaps as an experiment on the child's behalf, but if the notion about self is not revised, the individual is apt to resort to what is familiar. Thus a child fearful of school, who entertains notions about themselves as likely to panic if asked a question in class, is sorely tempted to avoid school. Such a child may develop a reasonably comprehensive view of life without school, and take to sleeping in on a morning, honing their knowledge of daytime television, and developing an expertise in deceiving parents.

Although the school refuser may be enticed back into school under threat or graduated exposure and support, the child may still retain a view of self as incompetent if asked questions in class. The anxiety faced by such a child, unsure of the possible implications regarding himself were he to have to answer questions, might maintain a sense of self as inept. In Kellyan terms, such a child experiences anxiety because the possible implications of failure – such as embarrassment, being thought of as foolish and so forth – are difficult to anticipate (lie outside the range of construing) as aspects of self construing. Therefore despite attending school, such a child with unresolved notions about publicly answering questions, is perhaps likely to revert to avoidance again.

Developing competence

Kelly chose to express his ideas somewhat abstractly, so his writings contain plenty of implications for clinical practice but precious few fully operationalised applications which might be straightforwardly transferred into work with children. This appears to have been no accident because Kelly point blank refused to provide sure-fire psychological remedies which might lure therapists into energetically treating their patients without going into the 'messy business' of understanding them first (Kelly 1969a).

In the context of accepting Kelly's suggestion of first enquiring why an individual wishes to change, before launching into techniques to promote change, a number of possible routes for increasing competence have been described:

- Develop notions about the desired behaviour. This might mean inviting the young person to describe in detail how he would ideally like to be. He might be asked to write a self characterisation as his ideal. He might be asked to observe or imagine someone who is competent in the area the child wishes to improve in. This might be followed up by pyramiding the described or identified characteristics in order that the intrinsic behaviours of such qualities are unearthed.
- A more formal methodology, consistent with the principles of personal construct theory, performance profiling (Butler and Hardy 1992; Butler 1996), encourages the individual to elicit the

qualities they consider necessary in order to perform well. This might be in social, artistic, scholastic or sporting endeavours. The individual then rates where they consider they are on each quality, perhaps using a 0–10 scale where a score of 10 represents the ideal. This exercise identifies areas the child feels they need to develop in order to perform well. The next step is to pinpoint pathways to achieving such qualities. This means specifying what to work on, or in Kellyan terms, what experiments to pursue.

- Identify experiments. This requires the child to generate ideas about how they might engage in actions that will improve their competence in a chosen area. It demands not only inspired notions of what they need to do, but a declared commitment to undertake such tasks and a willingness to examine their effects – authentic Kellyan experimentation in action.
- Constructively incorporate the results of an experiment with the individual's self construing. Should the child feel his actions are successful he might be encouraged to internalise his accomplishments. His competence is validated. A child might try cycling without stabilisers and survive without a grazed knee, or try informing his mother when upset rather than jumping out of the window and running away. Should the child sense their 'new' behaviour is successful then a re-evaluation of self is in order. The child might now consider himself to be something of a biker, or more adult in resolving their emotional problems respectively.

Fixed role therapy

A procedure which incorporates some of these ideas and one which Kelly most explicitly described, is fixed role therapy. This is a brief intervention in which the therapist and client jointly construct a specially tailored part for the client to play which will lead them into novel behavioural experiment, but not impel the individual to act out in a fashion that is either in total contradiction to their usual self or represents a brief excursion into their ideal way of functioning.

The case of Arthur describes how children may be encouraged to sample a different version of self and judge the implications of different actions (Green, 1997).

> Arthur was an 11-year-old boy. His mother, a single parent, had frequent contact with the Health Service for help in managing the severe behaviour problems presented by her youngest 5-year-old son Ben, who suffered from a range of developmental delays. She expressed a legitimate concern that Arthur would be adversely affected by being constantly asked to tolerate Ben's angry outbursts. Arthur, although much older than his brother, was described as being terrorised by his younger sibling and, in his mother's eyes, failing to assert himself appropriately in

the relationship. Although Arthur appeared to function reasonably well outside the family (e.g. with friends and at school), his mother feared his personality development might be impaired if he continued to be ruled by his handicapped brother.

Arthur acknowledged that he would like Ben to stop hitting him but did not share his mother's concern that being subjected to this regular pummelling would cause him long term psychological harm. He impressed as a gentle young man eager to please his mother and sensitive to the pressures under which she was struggling to bring up a family. The clinical challenge was to enable Arthur to try out new ways of coping with Ben's difficult conduct without instructing him to adopt a style grossly incongruent with his prevailing positive view of himself as a tolerant, considerate, kindly young man.

Arthur was asked to produce a self characterisation in which he wrote a brief pen-picture of himself described as if a character in a play. The account is written in the third person but is nonetheless an intimate and sympathetic portrayal of the important facets of the individual's personality. Arthur sketched himself thus:

> Arthur is an artistic boy. He likes P.E. and maths, but his favourite subject is art and craft. He is very trustworthy and gets along with people too. He wouldn't hurt a human or an animal, but he would try to defend himself if someone attacked him first. If he worked on a farm and had to kill a chicken or turkey for Christmas, he would probably refuse.
>
> He loves his family very much and knows what is right and wrong.
>
> Arthur is a bit shy when he talks to adults, because he thinks he might say something that the adult might not like.
>
> It is very important that his family is around him or near him.
>
> He used to have a Granny and Grandad but they died. They were nice people. They were his mother's parents.
>
> He enjoys going to his best friend's house. They go to the library and get some books out on things he is interested in. His friend is going to grammar school in September.
>
> It bothers him a little bit, but he hopes they still will be best friends.

In conversation, Arthur confirmed his view of himself as more of an Athenian than a Spartan who prided himself on his artistic gifts and sympathetic nature and had a strong aversion to violence no matter whether he was cast as the victim or aggressor. His sense of moral integrity and strong affection for his family also shone through. The overall tone of the self characterisation is hopeful rather than self critical and begins to explain why dealing with Ben's troublesome behaviour placed Arthur in something of a dilemma. How could he be true to himself and his values but nonetheless adopt a more determined and effective attitude towards his younger brother?

Arthur's mother also recognised that she wouldn't want him to change because 'he is a lovely lad who has a stream of nice qualities any mum would be proud to see in her son'. With Arthur's problems stemming from his tricky relationship with Ben the fixed role sketch was designed around a tight domestic 'mini-script' (Epting 1984).

The new identity Arthur was invited to adopt was that of Adam, whose character was typified as follows:

> *Adam is the sort of chap who likes to try and find solutions to problems. Sometimes answers come easily and it's good to know you've definitely got something right, but Adam also likes a challenge, and you can certainly call Ben a challenge.*
>
> *It's quite a trick to see some of Ben's antics as puzzles to be worked out but Adam is starting to get into the habit. Not that Adam always knows what to do – even Ben's mum is stumped by him sometimes. However, when there isn't a right thing to do, Adam just experiments and tries something new.*
>
> *Sometimes he's kind and understanding. Other times he takes no notice at all. Sometimes he gets upset and concerned. Other times he just doesn't give a damn. Sometimes he imagines he and his brother are two dinosaurs battling for survival. Other times he thinks of them as two co-stars in some epic film. He's decided that it is a good idea for now to keep Ben guessing and to become a bit more unpredictable.*
>
> *One of the things that allows Adam to take this relaxed 'suck it and see' approach is that he is very confident of his family's backing. Nobody is going to get seriously hurt so they trust his judgement. It's no big deal if things don't work out, and it's nice to get a bit of fun out of a situation that could get Adam down a bit if he let it.*
>
> *Above all, Adam likes to enjoy life and when he's happy he usually finds people around him are happy too. He finds he is at his most creative when he just follows his instincts and does what comes naturally. He likes to go his own way.*

The new part aimed to introduce Arthur to novel ways of reacting to Ben without asking him to adopt ways of construing himself that were in complete opposition to his prevailing self schema. Rather the introduction of the notion of Adam as a relaxed problem-solver tried to bring an unexpected and interesting fresh perspective to bear. In his role as Adam, Arthur might be freer to experiment in his dealings with Ben.

Arthur found Adam's character both acceptable and understandable and required little amendment. When asked how Adam's characteristics compared with his own personality, Arthur replied, after some reflection ... 'about half and half'. Such a common sense appraisal fits well with Kelly's more complex direction that the fixed role sketch should take an 'orthogonal' path in relation to the individual's dominant constructs regarding self.

As Kelly suggested, prior to enacting the new role, Arthur was asked to familiarise himself with the sketch, anticipate how Adam might react to Ben in various circumstances and briefly rehearse the role-play with his mother. He proved a convincing improviser and inventive and plausible actor. The enactment proper lasted 2 weeks and applied only to Arthur's conduct within home. He opted not to receive intensive support during the 2 weeks but asked that the therapist send him a postcard addressed to his *alter ego*, Adam. Following the enactment, Arthur attended the clinic with his mother to discuss how the experiment had gone and reflect on lessons learned.

Both Arthur's own report (through a diary log of his experiences) and his mother's contemporaneous observations confirmed that he enacted the Adam role faithfully and with an intriguing effect on Ben's conduct. While Adam was acting in a more relaxed and unpredictable fashion, Ben was reported to have become less aggressive and more respectful of his brother's wishes.

A further method, self appraisal profiling, was employed which enabled Arthur to describe himself on a limited number of personally important characteristics. This methodology, a simplified repertory grid, was originally developed to assist athletes to construe their performance and facilitate the coach's understanding of the athlete (Butler and Hardy 1992, Butler 1996). Arthur rated himself on nine constructs drawn from both his own self characterisation and Adam's fixed role sketch using a six-point scale. The constructs were:

- Gets along with people
- Relaxed
- Knows what's right and wrong
- Likes to enjoy himself
- Trustworthy
- Likes solving problems
- Would not hurt anyone
- Tries something new
- Loves his family.

Arthur's profile whilst undertaking the role of Adam (*Fig. 5.2*b) indicated he had a conceptual understanding of how the character differed from himself (*Fig. 5.2*a). As Adam he was more likely to try something new and be more relaxed.

It might have seemed the lessons to be drawn from the fixed role experiment were self evident. Of course, Arthur would conclude that his new repertoire of ways to manage Ben's difficult behaviour was both effective and personally comfortable and he would change accordingly. Arthur thought otherwise. He had listened closely to the terms of the experiment and understood correctly that he was to act 'as if' he were Adam for 2 weeks while his usual self was on a sort of brief

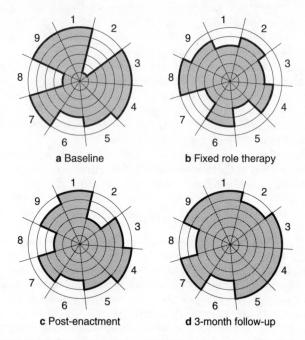

Fig. 5.2 Self descriptive profiles. 1, Gets along with people. 2, Relaxed. 3, Knows what's right and wrong. 4, Likes to enjoy himself. 5, Trustworthy. 6, Likes solving problems. 7, Would not hurt anyone. 8, Tries something new. 9, Loves his family

holiday. Following the enactment phase the old Arthur returned. He concluded that the fixed role had been very diverting but, upon reflection, had not led him to wish to redefine himself. He was quite happy with himself as he was.

Arthur's calm insistence on opting to retain his established version of himself is clearly portrayed in the post-enactment self appraisal profile (*Fig. 5.2*c) which closely resembles his baseline image. Not perhaps the 'good, rousing, construct-shaking experience' Kelly claimed fixed role therapy should provide, or so it appeared.

Arthur's mother feared he was putting a brave, public face on his private suffering and restated her continued concern that 'underneath' he was a sad and troubled young man. Arthur heard all this with a calm and unruffled dignity, appreciated his mother's viewpoint but sought to reassure her that he did truly hold a positive view of himself, his future and his capacity to deal constructively with Ben.

Three months later, during which Arthur moved from a small junior school to a large senior comprehensive school, a follow-up meeting brought evidence of a stunningly positive consensus. Arthur had coped with the school transfer in assured fashion and felt that, as he had predicted, he was managing Ben's behaviour to his satisfaction. Arthur's mother endorsed this change, describing his sense of buoyant self worth and how, during the school holiday, she had noticed Arthur reassuming some of the ways of coping with Ben that he had previously only employed in his fixed role persona of Adam. This was further highlighted by Arthur's self appraisal profile (*Fig. 5.2*d) with Arthur describing himself as much more relaxed and likely to try something new.

As much of the improvement appeared to lag behind the fixed role experience, coupled with the many other plausible and intervening positive influences in Arthur's life at the time, it would seem hazardous to claim that fixed role played a significant part in Arthur's increased confidence. On completion of the enactment phase of fixed role therapy, Arthur elected to reassume his former identity and run his life on familiar lines – as if nothing had happened. In personal construct terms choosing to define rather than extend one's construct system (to opt for an established way of viewing oneself rather than elaborating a new but risky perspective) is the preference of a person who feels better able to anticipate events from this position at this particular time. Arthur's candid resistance to further exploration of the implications of acting as if he were Adam can be seen as a healthy recognition that some of his core constructs of himself were under threat of imminent change, a process he was not about to rush into.

Kelly viewed creative problem-solving as an unending cycle of experiment and analysis, which he termed the loosening and tightening of the personal construct system. If fixed role therapy represents a carefully designed project to loosen existing constructs, then Arthur's immediately consequent choices can be seen as a timely tightening exercise. It is important however for this cycle to continue if the opportunity for change offered by the fixed role sketch is to be maintained. In terms of renewed behavioural experiment, Arthur's mother described how Arthur had acted in a more assertive manner towards Ben during the school holiday, feeling herself more relaxed about these brotherly exchanges and not impelled to intervene to protect Arthur. This picture resembled very similarly that reported during the fixed role enactment, only now it was Arthur, not Adam, who was centre stage.

The self appraisal profiles also provide evidence of continued reconstruing. The final profile (*Fig. 5.2*d) shows significant shifts from all three previous profiles. Arthur did not see himself as just like the Adam character he adopted during the fixed role enactment. It seems he found his own way of incorporating the qualities of being more relaxed and open to trying something new into his view of himself, whilst retaining those caring characteristics (such as being trustworthy and knowing what's right and wrong) that remained core to his identity. This appears to confirm Kelly's prediction that 'fixed role therapy is ... not a panacea but an experiment. In fact we have learned that if it is presented as a panacea it fails its purpose and the client does not get on with the process of finding out for himself' (Kelly 1969b).

Chapter 6
Children with troublesome behaviour

'The good bit about bedwetting is that it stops the dog sleeping on my bed'

'A person's behaviour is determined by the nature of their construct system' (Kelly 1970)

Kelly's construing of behaviour might be considered somewhat pre-emptive. However if, as Ravenette (1977) suggested, people do not appeal to their constructs in order to act, but rather they are their constructs, then Kelly's declaration makes convincing sense. If this hypothesis is extended and amplified so that problems are also considered to arise only from a person's construction of events, then we are faced with what Ravenette (1980) suggested is a 'tricky dilemma' when we seek to understand the behaviour problems of children.

Personal construct theory proposes fundamentally that individuals derive meaning through the way they construe the events they encounter. When a person cannot make sense of an event and feels that he should, then the person has a problem. Thus a child who wishes to have friends but who finds his approaches to others are unceasingly rebuffed, has a problem. His attempts to socialise, which reflect the child's notion of self as friendly, are exposed to serious invalidation. To avoid invalidation, the child might experience Kellyan hostility by denying he has any trouble with friendships and persistently seek out new relationships in ways that have already proved unfruitful.

Alternatively, the invalidation might generate Kellyan threat in that the child may begin to anticipate a revision or 'comprehensive change' of self construing which might lead the child to feel he is ultimately disagreeable, disliked and unsociable.

The problem arises not from the event itself, but from the child's inability to construe the event adequately, coupled with the feeling that he ought to be able to make sense of it. Children with so-called behaviour or conduct problems very rarely bemoan that they have a problem. Generally they are complained about. They are primarily problems to others, not to themselves. Their behaviour is troublesome because it impacts on other people – parents, teachers, neighbours and other children.

Children who are complained about

Ravenette (1988) sketched some customary gripes that adults have concerning children. They complain when they fail to understand the child and the child's way of conducting himself. Typically their efforts to anticipate the child's actions are met with disappointments, their attempts to unravel the puzzle of their behaviour met with frustration, their expectations defeated. The child becomes a threat to the adults' sense of 'knowingness'. The adult's construct system is expected to deal with events which lie outside its range of convenience, consequently experiencing what Kelly described as anxiety, being faced with a circumstance difficult to construe.

A second complaint Ravenette (1988) outlined alluded to the adult's sense of helplessness or incompetence. Adults complain when their efforts to alter the way the child is behaving fail to make any difference. Nothing they do seems able to influence what the child does. From a personal construct theory perspective it might be suggested that since the relationship between child and adult is proceeding far from smoothly, there is a failure in the adult's construction of the child's construing. As the sociality corollary predicts, when adults are faced with a child they find difficult to understand they may end up reacting to them, often in an authoritarian and intolerant manner, but primarily they fail to relate to them.

Behaviour which makes sense to the child

The complaint thus reveals who has the problem. Who is grappling to understand, striving and agonising over how to lessen the impact of the behaviour? For children their actions probably make perfect sense. What perplexes us about a behaviour may be completely understandable to the child.

Jackson and Bannister's (1985) intriguing study, briefly described in Chapter 4, emphasises this point. A group of children seen by their teachers as problematic and difficult were invited to discuss themselves, their troubles and relationships with the team of researchers. Fascinatingly Jackson and Bannister broadly discovered that most of the children perceived as difficult and incomprehensible made perfect sense of their own behaviour. It was as if, although perplexing and unintelligible to others, their actions made perfect sense to themselves.

The observer's perspective

Such findings expose a dilemma for clinicians who invest heavily in behaviour rating scales to assess the degree of abnormality of a child's behaviour. Almost without exception, such scales seek an opinion of the complainant, not the child complained about. Parents and teachers are asked to assess the child's behaviour as they perceive it. The scales illuminate nothing of the meaning of the behaviour. Thus a child might be construed as disturbed, maladjusted, and unbalanced because of how his actions are perceived, yet the child might perceive his own behaviour to be no more out of the ordinary than would the classically obedient child. As yet, few, if any, scales have yet been developed which tap the child's perception of their own behaviour. Personal construct theory offers the possibility of understanding what sense the child makes of his actions.

The child's perspective

Elaborating Kelly's theme that all actions are purposeful, Ravenette (1988) has compellingly offered an alternative to the conventional view of a behaviour being problematic. Taken from the child's standpoint he suggests we might persuasively ask for what problem is the behaviour a solution. Thus the child might be perceived as acting in a certain way because in doing so he resolves some other predicament.

It is hard to imagine that any child might find bedwetting a solution. Nevertheless studies which invite children to discuss what sense they make of the bedwetting have found, for a small number of children who wet the bed, this seems to be the case. Employing Tschudi's (1977) method of asking for the advantages and disadvantages of both the problem and perceived contrast, a few children volunteered advantages in continuing to remain wet at night. These were the very children who failed to respond to traditional interventions, indicating that indeed they may have found the enuresis to be a solution, rather than a problem.

Some of the perceived advantages of wetting included retaining a bedroom for themselves, avoiding having to sleep over at relatives, having the effect of stopping parents coming into the bedroom and 'telling me to tidy up', stopping the dog sleeping on the bed, and considering that the smell 'stops burglars breaking in' (Butler 1994; Butler et al. 1990). For such children the bedwetting would appear to be not so much a problem but a means to avoid facing perhaps a more difficult issue such as sharing a bedroom, staying over at a relatives, facing a nagging mother and so forth.

Behaviour as an expression of self construing

A list of childhood behaviours that adults complain about would be mind-bogglingly long. Some typical examples are lying, being cheeky, swearing, disrupting other children, calling names, graffiti, being cruel to animals, threatening others, stealing, fighting, breaking into other people's property, fire setting and vandalism.

Personal construct theory postulates that such behaviour is an expression of how the child construes himself and his world. If the child construes himself as a bully he will endeavour to find opportunities to taunt other children. Behaviour is further experimental in that the child is seeking to test out a prediction, so teasing a child younger than himself who recoils in tears, would validate the child's notion that taunting a young target is successful. The child's actions may further serve to confirm or define his notion of himself as a bully.

Such a child may subsequently seek to extend a notion of himself as powerful, dominant and forceful by acting in his intimidating manner towards other children or in other situations. Kelly (1955) described this – the individual's active elaboration – as aggressiveness. He was keen to define aggressiveness as what was going on inside the individual, not in terms of other people's reaction to the individual. Thus aggressiveness is the individual's active search to check out their construing, their search to widen the range of their understanding.

Thus the bully who seeks to extend his range of construing by taunting others on the rugby field might well come a cropper. He might give up on that experiment and alternatively test out being hard, disciplined or the perfect gentleman – all acts of Kellyan aggressiveness. Then again he might just decide to give rugby up altogether.

Behaviour as a stance

Behaviour however, is not always a question of observable movement. It may represent a particular stance, a viewpoint from which a lack of movement makes perfect sense to the child. A child's refusal to eat, listen, sleep, speak or go to school illustrate some examples. In a similar vein to how children's behaviour can be conceptualised, a child's refusal to act may also be seen as experimental, seeking validation and possibly the solution to some other problem. Butler (1985) for example described how a 12-year-old girl's refusal to attend school was best understood as the girl's frantic attempt to avoid separation from her parents, with a father about to embark on employment overseas and her mother recently starting work as a county councillor. The girl's school refusal appeared experimentally to be testing the parents' decisions about their employment and ultimately to protect (or solve for her) her sense of vulnerability.

Children referred for behaviour problems

The case of Gary might further elaborate some of the issues concerning children complained about because of behavioural problems. Gary was 11 years old when referred by his GP. He was the middle of three children, all close in age. His elder sister was described as very bright intellectually and thriving at school. His brother, just a year younger, was excelling at sport, both at school and at a local club. Gary's mother was white and his father a black South African, and they were bringing the children up within a nuclear family unit.

Gary's mother frankly but compassionately expressed her concerns. Gary was involved in a wide range of behaviours that she found baffling and she felt despondently incapable and powerless to change his conduct. Gary was sniffing petrol, aerosols, deodorants and butane gas, smoking regularly, breaking into premises – shops and houses – stealing (for which he was already on conditional discharge) and taking vehicles.

Gary's parents tried to intervene by grounding him, and at their wits' end, had stopped him going on a rugby tour with the club he played for. This served only to escalate the tension between Gary and his parents. In seeking to understand the mordancy Gary described how he felt his mother lacked trust in him and that she was ashamed of him. Further, Gary surmised that when his mother quizzed him about his behaviour, this afforded more evidence that he was not to be trusted and validated her opinion that he had let them down. Sport seemed to be one area where Gary shone. He was stocky and well built, ideal for rugby, and his other passion, boxing. The Self Image Profile (*Table 6.1*) displays this with a maximum rating.

Gary's Self Image Profile shows him to have a positive regard for himself. He construes himself as helpful, sporting and is pleased with his appearance. His sociability is manifest by high ratings on making friends easily, helpfulness and being good fun coupled with low ratings on loneliness and shyness. Gary reveals a sense of feeling different from others, which he considered was the upshot of his colour and the consequent gibes and provocation from others.

The profile additionally displays Gary's negative view of himself. He regarded himself as inclined to argue (with his sister, mother and teacher), stubborn, cheeky, bad tempered, easily bored (especially at school) and always in trouble. A hint at Gary's predicament was

Table 6.1 Gary's Self Image Profile

How would you describe yourself?	Not at all						Very much so
	0	1	2	3	4	5	6
Kind					▨		●
Make friends easily							▨●
Well liked						▨	●
Good fun						▨	●
Lots of energy							▨●
Helpful							▨●
Honest				▨			●
Good at sport							▨●
Intelligent/smart					▨		●
Like the way I look							▨●
Feel different from others	●				▨		
Lazy	●					▨	
Lonely	▨●						
Stubborn	●						▨
Moody			●	▨			
Always in trouble	●				▨		
Shy	▨●						
Cheeky	●					▨	
Argue a lot	●						▨
Bad tempered	●						▨
Get bored easily	●						▨

▨ 'as I am'; ● 'as I'd like to be'.

revealed in his account of why he was always in trouble, when he described how he was unable to say 'no' when egged on by others.

Gary was further invited to make a rating of how he would ideally like to be. In *Table 6.1* his observations, particularly on negative descriptions, were mostly at the extreme and as such represent something of a fantasy. As Kelly (1955) indicated, an alternative to the problem although available, may be unrealistically drawn and over-simplified. How Gary would like to be seemed a distant, almost

unobtainable vision, a vision which may have, by its contrast, corro-
borated Gary's perception of self as 'antisocial'.

Having recently moved to high school Gary was struggling to settle.
He was described as disruptive and willingly volunteered his resistance
to doing any homework. Gary's explanations hinged around a conviction that other children on his table prevented him working, an acute
nervousness about having to read in class and his experiences of
finding written work laborious, uninviting and difficult. An assessment
of Gary's level of cognitive functioning subsequently revealed no
obvious areas of anomalous or unusual performance other than a slight
difficulty with spelling.

Eliciting constructs

Out of school, partly because of his thickset appearance, Gary chose to
spend time with boys older than himself. From a list of peers both from
within school and outside of school Gary described how he was both
similar and different from these friends. By seeking the contrasts of the
elicited descriptions, a series of constructs were derived. These are
arranged below. Gary perceived himself to be on the left hand side of
each of the constructs:

Likes to go out	Boring
Likes sport	Boring
Bad tempered	Kind of shy
Shows off when with friends	Shy
Can't say no	Can say no
Messes about	Does work/listens to teacher
If dared, he'd do it	Too serious
Has fun	Serious

The implications of constructs

Gary was able to appreciate both how his notions about himself led him
into constantly being in trouble and how the implications of the contrast
states made it hazardous to change. Not to be in trouble would imply
for Gary a state of seriousness and boredom. Gary further elaborated
this notion of himself as always being in trouble, being unable to say no
and eager to accept a dare by reflecting on the advantages such
behaviour accrued to him. Asking for advantages of the present state
and disadvantages of a contrast state, according to Tschudi (1977),
highlights the dilemma facing the individual.

Without hesitation, Gary intimated that the advantage of showing
off, undertaking dares and so on, was the attention he received. He

described how you get a 'name', become known as someone not to be messed with, and avoid being called a chicken or wimp. The disadvantages of refusing a dare were that 'you might not be part of the group', face being called chicken and get called 'paki'. Such powerful implications of the contrast tend to maintain the individual's course of action. Change would be perceived as hazardous at best.

Gary appeared to seek validation from his peers. He successfully experienced acceptance and recognition through his behaviour. Most individuals strive to be recognised rather than remain anonymous. Gary would rather have a 'name' than be a nobody, or worse still be known as a 'paki'. Personal construct theory suggests all behaviour is legitimate and meaningful. Understanding Gary's perspective bears this out.

Behaviour as an experiment

As discussed previously, personal construct theory persuades us to consider behaviour as an experiment. This subtle invitation dramatically presents a positive reframing to what others might perceive as a problem. Kelly (1970) suggested that behaviour is man's principal instrument of inquiry. Our actions test out our hypotheses. We test our predictions about how things might turn out. We strive to create meaning and certainty. Our actions validate aspects of ourselves. We may enact new behaviours in thrashing around for a fresh identity.

Gary's behaviour was undoubtedly persistent. It had brought him face to face with the police on at least two occasions, dogged complaints from school and enduring appeals from his parents for help. Whilst his actions made perfect sense to Gary, validating his notion of self, he was in danger of serious trouble and exclusion from school should they persist.

Invitation to change

What, however, were the avenues of change? The contrast to his construing looked a bleak and uninviting option for Gary. In his usual perceptive way, Kelly (1955) had discussed how clients' and parents' complaints are usually 'poorly formulated' in the sense that they rarely open up avenues to a happy solution. He was however a keen advocate of listening to the complaint, and of seeking to understand it, which he argued helped establish rapport through attending to areas which the complainant considered important. Kelly (1970) further offered a teasing possibility. He suggested that if a person endlessly repeats the same behaviour then 'I shall suspect he is still looking for the answer to a question he knows no better way of asking'. Could Gary find better or alternative ways of asking his questions?

Ravenette (1977) has argued that the most important tool the therapist has in helping children to discover new behaviours and make, as it were, renewed enquiries, is the question. Ravenette's rule of thumb in asking questions of children are:

- Ask for three responses: this implies for the child that there are no right or wrong answers.
- Never ask 'why?': children are forever being asked why they did this or that and it is therefore usually interpreted by the child as threatening. It is perhaps better to ask 'how come?'
- Seek the contrast: helping children elaborate the contrast to their construing enhances an understanding of the child's meaning.
- Go along with what the child says but be prepared to clarify and challenge what he says in the pursuit of greater understanding.

Self creation

In seeking fresh options for Gary, Kelly, as so often, provides a starting point. In much of what he discussed about individuals being experimenters and creators of their own worlds, he invites us to extend this capacity to invent ourselves anew and change what we do not like about ourselves. Therapy might thus be construed as self creation, not self correction (Neimeyer and Harter 1988). Dalton and Dunnett (1992) suggest that if all our present interpretations of the universe are subject to revision or replacement then this must include our interpretations of ourselves. Laudable intentions but what of an individual, like Gary, who didn't reckon much to the idea of change?

Perhaps therapy, as Epting (1984) suggested, has to become something of a 'playful enterprise'. Gary would have to be coaxed into considering change. If we search sweepingly, avenues of possible change can surprisingly appear. The Self Image Profile is often an enticing start. A survey of Gary's Self Image Profile (*Table 6.1*) shows the extent of the discrepancy between self and ideal. Such discrepancies have customarily, within personal construct theory, been employed as a measure of self esteem. A small discrepancy suggests a high self esteem; a large discrepancy suggests low self esteem.

Reducing the discrepancy between self and ideal has therefore been suggested as a means of increasing self esteem. With the birth of psychology, William James (1892) suggested that a re-examination or reconstruing of the ideal self may be as appropriate a therapeutic goal as reconstruing the actual self. However such 'downgrading' of the ideal self from fantasy to reality has the danger of reducing the child's aspirations. Do we really want to shatter children's dreams of scoring the winner at Wembley or being a Hollywood star?

Selecting areas of potential change

Rather than focus on those aspects of the Self Image Profile where there were large discrepancies between Gary's vision of self and ideal, he was cautiously asked to mull over two aspects where the discrepancy was not so great – 'kind' and 'always in trouble'. His profile suggested there were times when he was kind and not in trouble. He was thus asked to describe those times. To illustrate with examples, what he would be engaged in when he was kind and not in trouble. Seeking behavioural descriptors of constructs in this way, as described in Chapter 2, is a form of pyramiding (Fransella and Dalton 1990).

Gary said he was kind when he cleaned up at home. As for when he was not in trouble, Gary elaborated this in three ways. He was not in trouble when:

1. Playing sport – boxing, running, rugby and athletics,
2. Doing practical work such as fixing things like his bike, which also relieved boredom, and
3. When he tackled an interesting project at school and the teacher told him he had done well.

When engaged in these ways Gary said it made him feel good and gave him a sense of achievement.

Reconstruction

Winter (1992) has suggested that only those interventions which offer the child the possibility of further extension or definition of the construct system can be expected to lead to reconstruction. In asking Gary to attend to exceptions it might serve to hint at possible ways of changing. Further, in inviting Gary to describe his feelings (good) and implications (achievement) of the 'exceptions' – those times he behaves in ways that are not typical of the complaint – the intention was both to elaborate these experiences and foster a definition of himself as someone 'not always in trouble'.

Seeking exceptions in this way, and harnessing an understanding of what might account for the exceptions, can be a powerful means of re-creation. When undertaken in the presence of the complainant – parent or teacher – at the very least it enables them to consider the problem as transient and the child as possibly responsive, and hopefully it may secure a shift in their perception of the child, and thus enhance the opportunity of them recognising the child's changed behaviour, which in turn validates the child's reformulated vision of self.

Elaborating the contrast

In seeking to enhance Gary's vision of himself as kind and not always in trouble there was an intention, as eloquently expressed by Fransella (1972) to 'locate the self in the contrast'. To, as it were, dismantle Gary's way of life (as always in trouble) and seek to increase or develop the implications for constructs which form a new way of life. Fransella (1972), in her work with stutterers, found that unless she developed the individual's vision of self as fluent (the contrast to stuttering) through encouraging experimentation with fluency then the child was forever vulnerable to stuttering.

Facilitating a change in behaviour may be reasonably straightforward, but securing a more permanent change will only occur once the individual comes to see the new behaviour as representative of himself. Thus so long as Fransella's stutterers perceived themselves as stutterers, no matter how fluent they were, they would revert on occasions to stuttering. The hazardous task in the process of change is not so much supporting the individual in making the changes but in fostering a revision of self, so the person feels the new behaviour fits with their vision of self.

Salmon (1995) has made a similar point in her description of the learning process. She contended that as all learning has implications, there is a Kellyan choice in whether an individual will embark on learning anything new. If it defines or extends the vision of self the person may embark willingly on new ventures. Thus connoisseurs have a healthy appetite to learn new skills in areas in which they are expert. Thus Gary might willingly venture into antisocial behaviours which extend his notion of troublesome behaviour and hone a definition of 'always in trouble'. Salmon further argued that as knowledge is not 'free-standing or disembodied', particular spheres of knowing 'belong' – to particular concerns and particular lifestyles. Thus learning a musical instrument or understanding opera might not be an option to someone who conceives of himself as 'tone deaf', not because he hasn't the capacity to learn, but because the individual perceives himself as unmusical in these areas.

Such ideas alert us to the importance of working within the child's construct system. Only through understanding the child's sense of self, his mode of construing and the implications of change for the child can he be encouraged to explore different behaviour. Too often, in our eagerness to help, we fail to respect the constraints imposed by the structures in which the child currently lives (Neimeyer and Harter 1988).

Kelly's ideas of change were discussed in Chapter 2. They all emphasise the restructuring of the child's own current constructions. This serves again to emphasise the impotency of 'off the shelf' solutions and glib reassurance or advice.

Observing others

Staying with the thesis of considering change from the client's perspective, another powerful means of controlled elaboration is asking the child to, as it were, become an observer. Gary was asked about other children who sometimes got into trouble, got dared to do things they knew were troublesome and messed about, and invited to observe how they dealt with such situations differently from how he might typically act. Winter (1992) has suggested that by engaging clients in this way they may come to consider the complaint within socially shared, rather than purely personal dimensions, and that if they are able to view the complaint as if it were someone else's, then reconstruction might appear less threatening.

Gary identified one boy in his class at school who generally kept himself out of trouble. Gary described him as 'in control'. In pyramiding again (asking Gary to describe what the boy did when he showed he was in control) Gary said the boy would do what he wanted, not what other kids dared him to do; he would laugh off any taunts; walk away from any jibes; he listened in class; he would ask the teachers for help when he got stuck. This was a fairly thorough elaboration of the contrast.

Asking Gary to describe how he felt this boy was able to conduct himself in this way, he reckoned the boy would be cool and he would think others who called him a wimp would be thick and stupid. A follow-up question sought to understand how Gary might feel if he were able to be like this boy. Without a hint of hesitation Gary said that for him to act like this boy would mean he would 'feel like I've turned a corner'.

Inviting new experimentation

Gary was asked if he could imagine himself undertaking any of these alternative courses of action. He reckoned he could laugh off the taunts and dares of others. In class he felt able to ask the teacher when he got stuck. Here the aim was to attempt to design an experiment for Gary to test outside the therapy room. Gary was being invited to approach familiar situations as if some new construction reflected his vision of self.

The invite to act *as if* is an especially valued approach in personal construct theory. In its most formal state it has been scripted into fixed role therapy and described fully in Chapter 5. More usually it takes the form of an invitation to the child to enact an experiment, to act in a planned alternative way. Winter (1992) has argued that such experimentation enables the child to 'disengage core constructs from the experimentation by seeing it as only acting a point'. Any threat which the 'new' behaviour might normally evoke by virtue of its inconsistency with core structures is therefore minimised.

A remarkable study illustrating the potency of *as if* experimentation is found in a study undertaken by Robert Hartley (1986). He asked a group of 7- and 8-year-old children to undertake a matching task twice, and on the second occasion they were encouraged to complete it *as if* they were someone very clever. Children who 'as themselves' had completed the task impulsively, engaged in the task much more vigilantly, accurately and diligently when they responded as if they were clever. Such results indicate that even such supposedly inflexible and rigid attributes as cognitive functioning may be the product of roles we inhabit. With some creativity these children showed the potential for changing the way they were, by reinventing themselves (although only for the duration of the experiment), and what's more they devised some appropriate behaviours to bring it about.

Emotional implications of change

The emotional implications of change have to be anticipated. Kelly defined emotional experiences as the consequence of constructs in transition. Any change in construing might therefore be expected to result in some degree of anxiety, threat or guilt. The adoption of a changed way of acting or reconstruction might only occur if the anticipated change or change itself does not confront the child with too high a degree of anxiety, threat or guilt. If experiences encountered by the changed behaviour are too discrepant from existing constructs, then Kellyan anxiety is provoked. Anxiety is the awareness of stark unpredictability.

If the person becomes aware of an impending change in their sense of self that is inconsistent with their core role structures (their vision of self) then threat is experienced. Threat is the awareness of radical inconsistency. If a person recognises they are acting or likely to act in ways they would not have predicted in themselves then they experience guilt. Guilt might be construed as the awareness of specific dislodgement.

Engaging in new experiments

Having explored some alternatives for Gary, he was asked to try to imagine himself in various scenarios – being dared to do things that he knew would lead him into trouble; struggling with some work at school – and to picture in 'his mind's eye' his new, alternative ways of responding. Once able to do this Gary was asked to try it out, to act as if he were the sort of person who took control by laughing off ridicule, provocation and baiting, and seeking help with class projects when stuck, for 2 weeks. Imagination and enactment facilitate reconstruing by tempering the emergence of emotional responses, a playful enterprise indeed.

However before embarking upon the new role, Gary's mother, who had been present throughout, was invited to contribute to Gary's new venture. In facilitating mother's understanding of Gary's viewpoint and his imminent experiment it was hoped that both the mother's sense of 'knowingness' would increase (thus reducing her complaints of an inability to comprehend) and that there would be an increased chance that Gary's new ventures and adopted construing would be validated outside the therapy room. In tightening up her responses to Gary she agreed:

1. Not to shout but listen to Gary's version of events.
2. To be clear with Gary about what was expected of him, so that any reversion to former behaviour would be met with a reminder of what it was he had agreed to try out.
3. To be positive, not looking for when things went wrong but searching out and recognising the efforts Gary made to maintain his experimental behaviours.

Gary returned 2 weeks later in jubilant mood. He described some successes in laughing off the exhortations to mess about in class, although the baiting by his peers, if anything, he sensed had increased. He was able to construe his persistent experimenting in the face of such pressures to succumb, as further evidence of his resilience to persist and 'take control'. He was most eager to tell of his success in class where his endeavours to listen and seek help had resulted in the achievement of a merit. Interestingly Gary had also begun to make some decisions about developing his sporting talent to a greater extent. He had been to rugby training sessions regularly, begun to mix more with other players and had been picked for the first time to captain the team in a competitive match the next weekend. It was tempting to ask if Gary had endeavoured to elaborate his new construing in a different context – rugby – from that which we had originally set out. However, instead, his enthusiasm for this new venture was harnessed by seeking to discover what it was that he had changed about his approach to rugby, with a view of possibly engaging this construing in other aspects of his life.

Gary eagerly talked of how he approached his game and what was expected of him. He described the need for discipline, the need to follow the coach's instructions, the need to support others on the field, the need for nerves of steel in tackling and so forth. All of these attributes Gary noticed were possible to apply to other settings, both when out with his friends and within school. A second experiment was suggested, whereby Gary would endeavour to apply his sporting self to the rigours of school and the harassment of peers; a further version of the *as if* approach. Mair (1977a) has noted how the use of a metaphor like this can facilitate an elaboration of construing and experimentation. Gary was undoubtedly ready to have a go with this experiment.

Conclusion

Children's behaviour is often a source of concern. There is a sense, within society, that children's behaviour is becoming worse. Most referrals to general child psychology and psychiatry services consist of complaints about behaviour, framed in terms of disturbance, non-compliance, aggressiveness and being 'out of control'. When it comes to their behaviour, it seems children are complained about, but rarely complain themselves.

A personal construct perspective implies that the child's behaviour, however perplexing to the complainant, makes sense to the child. The child's actions are experiments, ways of testing out their construct system. As the example of Gary illustrates, the changes other people – parents, teachers and society in general – might expect or wish for, in a young person's behaviour, will only occur if the change makes sense to the individual. The task for those who wish to foster change in children's behaviour is to find ways of engaging and guiding them towards more 'socially appropriate' experiments, but ones that do not pose a threat to the child.

Chapter 7

Children in trouble with the law

'It just seemed like a bit of fun'

August bank holiday Monday. The drought of that summer stretched on. Three boys woke to a cloudless, sun baked morning. Another sweltering long day stretched in front of them. A day to be filled with amusement, recreation, horseplay, and a dash of devilment. One to be anticipated with some relish. No different to the start of many other days that had characterised the extended school holiday. Except that this would end with the death of an elderly lady and one of the boys – a mere 10 years old – charged with murder. What had seemed like just a bit of fun had dramatically, in seconds, veered alarmingly into a nightmare.

The police records provide a summary of that fateful day. John, along with Alan and Carl 'tricked' their way into a high rise block of flats, as they had done on a number of previous occasions. Once inside the building they made their way on to the roof, through a vandalised door. The flat roof provided a spectacular view across the busy city. But the 10-year-old boys were not necessarily taken in by the panorama. Besides they had been there before. They were experimenters, doers, interested in action and thrills. Before long the boys found an orange and then a piece of wood, which were both propelled over the 5 foot parapet to the ground below.

Escalation seems fundamental to play; taking a theme and amplifying, intensifying, expanding as the child's involvement grows. In such vein a discarded piece of concrete weighing almost 20 lbs was heaved up and placed on the parapet, a parapet some 2 inches higher than John's height. John admitted later, to the police, that he was responsible for pushing the concrete block over the edge. Directly below, unseen by John, stood a group of people returning from the shop, via the back entrance, to the block of flats. The concrete block hit, and instantly killed one of them, an elderly lady. The boys fled the scene and were, within an hour, picked up by the police.

Legal framework

After admitting responsibility, John was legally described under the terms of the Child and Young Persons Act 1953 as *doli incapax*. This Act states that children under 10 years cannot be found guilty of an offence, and that children between 10 and 14 years are presumed to be incapable of forming criminal intent. In order that John might therefore be tried, the Crown Prosecution Service had to counter the presumption of *doli incapax*. It had to seek to demonstrate that John knew or understood the difference between right and wrong, and was aware at the time that he was acting in a way that was seriously wrong, in contrast to what might otherwise be construed as naughty or mischievous.

Determining a child's awareness of the 'wrongness' of an act he is engaged in has proved to be a hazardous business. The behaviour itself cannot be presented as evidence to prove a child knows right from wrong because the immediate repercussions of the behaviour (such as arrest) may affect the child's judgement retrospectively about the seriousness of the act. Neither can the child's reactions following the behaviour be used to demonstrate that, at the time, he knew he was engaged in behaviour which was seriously wrong. For example, running away from the scene cannot be used to judge the wrongness of the act, because children customarily tend to escape from commonplace and petty acts of mischievousness.

The legal question of ascertaining whether John knew at the time of pushing the block off the roof, that he was engaged in an act that could be considered seriously wrong, is identical to that placed before Bobby Thompson and Jon Venables, the boys found guilty of abducting 2-year-old James Bulger and killing him on a railway line in 1993. In that case the Crown Prosecution Service requested a psychiatric opinion to determine if there was a case of 'diminished responsibility' and a clinical psychologist to assist in the assessment of moral understanding. Only Jon Venables agreed to be seen, although at a very late stage with the weight of forensic evidence against him, Bobby Thompson agreed to see a child and adolescent psychiatrist appointed by the defence, but refused to see the psychiatrist for the Crown.

Assessment

John was seen within 6 weeks of the fateful day. It was explained that the purpose of seeing a psychologist was to seek to understand how it was that he had arrived in this predicament and that a report of the interview and assessments would subsequently be written for the Court. There was undoubtedly some anticipated unease concerning the troublesome task of harmonising psychological information with what can appear to be a rigid legal framework.

On first meeting John, Kelly's first principle of finding out – that of asking the client – was considered perhaps not to be the most apposite strategy in ascertaining his version of the event. After all John was not seeking the resolution to a problem in the way Kelly had in mind in his appeal for personal inquiry. John had not been brought kicking and screaming, but because the system demanded it. It was therefore considered more appropriate to ask about the events on the roof at the very end of our two sessions. Even though John would communicate unreservedly about many things during the sessions, often with a flash of humour, he resurrected a tight lipped, avoidant posture to any 'awkward' questions. Interestingly this bears a resemblance to Jon Venables who also reportedly became subdued and uncommunicative when asked about the charges by the psychologist (Smith 1994).

'Mental normality' has in practice often been accepted as proof of a child's ability to distinguish right from wrong. The contrast suggests that a child who demonstrates bizarre or 'abnormal' development cannot be held accountable for his behaviour and would therefore be described as *doli incapax* on the grounds of diminished responsibility. There seemed little evidence to suggest John's mental development was abnormal. His mother described him as a normal cheeky boy 'in common with others of his age', with a tendency to resort to swearing and an inclination to play with mischievous boys, sometimes younger than himself. John's mother blamed her partner, whom she described as 'a really foul mouthed person when drunk'. John's favourite TV programmes were World Wrestling, Bart Simpson and the Power Rangers. If he were a Power Ranger he said he would be able to fly and do somersaults in the air. John fully recognised this made them different from himself, and as some might argue, demonstrated a differentiation of reality from fantasy. Interestingly he struggled to find any difference between himself and Bart Simpson, primarily, indeed exclusively, because the character was construed in terms of always being in trouble. John perceived an affinity with Bart Simpson through their shared infringements of parental and societal expectations.

A child's level of intellectual capacity has also been linked, perhaps understandably, although not always logically, with the child's capacity to distinguish right from wrong. There was little doubt that John's level of cognitive development, assessed on the British Ability Scales (BAS), was within a 'normal range', although at the lower end of this range. Interestingly this placed John's intellectual capacity on the very boundary where the law absolves the child of responsibility. Thus the Children and Young Persons Act 1953 regards children under 10 years (chronological not intellectual) as *doli incapax* and unable to be found guilty of an offence.

What, however, also emerged from the assessment of cognitive functioning and attainment tasks was clear evidence of a specific learning difficulty. John, it turned out, was profoundly affected by dyslexia. Both his decoding (reading) skills and encoding (spelling) ability were estimated to be around the 6 to 6.6 year level, so ill-developed that his scores lay beyond the range of the centile scales. For example, John read 'here' for her, 'can' for cup, 'did' for bird and 'pig' for dig. He attempted only eight words on the BAS spelling test, with 'mi' being his attempt at 'my', and 'yu' for 'up'.

A delineation of dyslexia demands primarily that there is a significant discrepancy between the level of intellectual functioning and level of reading (Rutter and Yule 1975). Tables in which reading achievement is predicted on the basis of the observed correlations between educational attainment, age and intellectual level in the general population offer the most appropriate means of understanding the degree of underachievement (Rutter and Yule 1979). According to tables published by the BAS (Elliott 1983), only 1% of children would have a discrepancy as large as John's between reading level and what would be expected given his level of intellectual functioning. The experience of struggling with dyslexia can be traumatic. Of relevance here, however, is how such a specific difficulty might have played a part in John's plight. Noticeably, perhaps significantly, John's dyslexia had gone unnoticed at school. A Statement of Special Educational Needs, designed chiefly to emphasise John's behavioural difficulties, made reference to literacy difficulties in passing, but no specific or focused help for John's dyslexia had ever been envisaged.

Run of the mill implications of dyslexia include the difficulty of assimilating and processing information in both the verbal and visual modality, and an inability to think through or analyse all the possible consequences of any behaviour (Rutter and Yule 1979). Children with dyslexia may therefore neglect to take things into account before acting. Kelly might have considered this as a shortening of the circumspection–pre-emption–control (CPC) cycle where the child omits to consider all the information (lacking circumspection), but elects to act pre-emptively and perhaps impulsively in relating to events before him.

The very nature of John's dyslexia may thus counter the notion that he knew at the time of the incident that he was engaged in a behaviour which was seriously wrong. It could be argued that he would have struggled to weigh up or predict the ramifications and thus the entire risk of his action, particularly as he was prevented, by the height of the parapet, of gathering information about what was below. Nevertheless the prosecution would argue that John's two companions, keeping an eye out for what was happening below, shouted to him not to do it. What the boys actually shouted, the intention behind their cries and John's possible interpretation of this remains open to question. What seems crucial is not what was said, but what meaning John attached to it. It is of course commonplace that we read other people's intentions wrongly. We can easily misinterpret other people's meaning. When a mother eventually gives in to the toddler's request for a biscuit, do all her earlier 'no's', from the child's perspective really mean 'yes'?

The issue of misinterpretation has perhaps never been more powerfully exhibited, in British criminal circles, than in the case of Derek Bentley. In 1952, Bentley, along with another youth, Christopher Craig, set out one November evening looking for excitement. Their thoughts turned to the possibility of robbing a store in Croydon, and with this in mind they climbed on the roof of a warehouse building. Soon they were confronted by the police. Bentley, aged 19, and who suffered with a 'low IQ', a reading age of between 4 and 5 years and a history of epilepsy, was quickly apprehended. Craig, aged 16, then pulled a gun. It is alleged Bentley, who was already under arrest, shouted, 'Let him have it Chris' to the other boy who then shot and killed one of the policemen. Bentley said he meant it as an instruction to surrender the gun. The prosecution, at his trial, argued that Craig had interpreted the comment as an instruction to shoot. Both were found guilty of murder under the ancient doctrine of 'constructive malice'. Because of his age, Craig was sentenced to be detained at Her Majesty's pleasure and served his time in Wakefield Jail. Bentley, being of an age of criminal responsibility, went to the gallows. He remains the only accomplice to a capital crime ever to be executed when the principal had, for reasons of youth or insanity, escaped the death penalty.

Understanding John's dilemma

Rutter and Yule (1979) amongst others have described how dyslexia can have a profound effect on a child's behaviour, self worth and social development. These three phenomena play a vital part in understanding John's dilemma.

Behaviour

John's behaviour, particularly at school, had been in the spotlight for some time. Following the Bulger case where the boys' school teachers gave evidence both on the school's philosophy – the importance of teaching children to behave responsibly towards one another – and specific teaching of right and wrong, it was natural that John's teachers would be asked to comment. The evidence of two of John's most recent teachers outlined a weighty history of wrongdoing and their sustained efforts to teach the difference between right and wrong.

The teachers' endeavours in seeking to raise an awareness of what was acceptable and unacceptable behaviour led to an assertion that John had indeed been taught to understand what was wrong. However, a complication arises when a child who has been taught to understand wrongness continues to act in ways that are seen to be wrong, as John had done. It might be considered that the moral teaching failed to be taken in by the child. A difficulty in assimilating information, a root attribute of dyslexia, might plausibly have impeded John's access to such teaching. What is under question here is the degree to which what is taught is correlated with what is learnt. Alternatively a child might continue to act in inappropriate ways despite moral teaching because the child chooses to, as it were, to ignore what is taught. Thus a child may have a fair grasp of the concept of wrongness, but still choose to act in ways that are considered wrong. Knowledge and action might therefore fail to be correlated. This issue is at the core of countering the presumption of *doli incapax*.

Herein lies the problem for teachers. They typically tend to construe children from the outside, looking in. They adopt an observer's perspective. However comprehensive and accurate that perception is, it is nevertheless a view, a construction of the child, based on a framework that makes sense to them. An observer's attribution of a problem is generally marked by a constitutional belief. We reason that a child behaves as they do because of something (wrong) about them. This generally contrasts with the actor's perspective, the person engaged in the behaviour. They tend to attribute the reason for their behaviour in situational terms. The particular circumstances at the time are seen to be contributory. In seeking the 'inside version', the child's perception of events, a teacher might take the opportunity to try Kelly's first principle on for size. This suggests that if we wish to know why a child persists in behaving in troublesome ways, it might prove fruitful to ask about their version of events. As Ravenette (1977) proposed so clearly, gathering an awareness of the child's troubles can be assisted greatly by going beyond the traditional grasp of understanding (the observer's perspective) and seeking to understand the child's understanding.

An extensive 'behavioural log' was kept by the teachers for a 12-week period in the autumn of the school year which saw John first excluded from the school, enter a special school and conclude with a charge of murder against him. *Table 7.1* is a summarised representation of that behaviour log. It represents the contrasting statements made by John's teacher and presents a framework to resemble a series of

Table 7.1 A summary of teachers' construing of John, from the behaviour log

A	B
1. Concentrates	Bored
2. Sit quietly	Singing; muttering; talk loudly; noisy making silly baby noises loudly; swearing; banging legs on desk
3. Sit in own place	Moved around carpet; leaving seat; fidgeted around classroom
4. Settle	Disruptive; telling tales; show off
5. Ask advice; listen to my opinion	Ignore me; cheeky parrot towards me; mimic me
6. Co-operate (do what I ask)	Flatly refused; ignored
7. Worked well; worked hard	Wouldn't work; refused to do work
8. Work with others (collaborate)	Prevented others working
9. Join in; offer suggestions; take turns	Sit on own; standing out; refuse to join in
10. Worked with a partner; worked well together	Chatting loudly to them; mocked others; hit others; teasing; taunting; incited; saying unkind things to others; tried to annoy others; punched; insulted; threw conkers at others

constructs. The fascinating insights generated by this are many fold, but the broad outcome reflects Kelly's view that explanations offered about children's actions often tell us more about the construct system of the adult than the child. The more 'acceptable' end of the construct is arranged on the left side, under A, and the unwelcome or undesirable pole on the right side, under B.

The constructs have a time-honoured pedagogic flavour. John was expected to conform to traditional educational values: concentrating on task, constrained to his seat, showing respect and submissiveness to authority, putting effort into his work and working constructively alongside or with other children. The agenda was fixed. John was to be moulded into what school expected of him. There was little leeway. Sadly missing was any consideration of John's perceived needs.

Tellingly, the behavioural log indicated that John was at various times located at both poles of every construct. Sometimes he worked well, and at other times he refused to work. Occasionally he joined in with others and offered helpful suggestions yet at other times he sat on his own away from the group. From time to time he would listen to the teacher and then he would mimic and 'parrot' her. From the teacher's perspective John would seem to slot rattle – vacillate rapidly between the two opposing poles of a construct. Kelly argued that shifting between poles of a construct in this way represents the least stable form of change (Winter 1992). The behaviour log reported that John 'can only be good for so long'. Essentially John perplexed the teachers. They could not readily predict his behaviour.

From John's perspective he might have felt misunderstood. He might be seen as actively testing out, like the scientist Kelly postulated, the strangulating system within which he was being expected to function. Kelly considered this might be viewed as aggressiveness – the vigorous elaboration of one's perceptual field. Kelly aspired to be non-judgemental about such experimenting, seeing it as the individual's search for validity, although from an observer's point of view suffering the effects, John's spirited elaboration might well have been a disturbing experience.

Of further note, *Table. 7.1* illustrates that John was mostly located at the troublesome end of the constructs (B). He was construed, mostly, as contravening appropriate school behaviour, to the point whereby transgressions might have been predicted as the norm for John. He was expected to misbehave, and any such acts would serve to validate the teachers' view of John. From the behaviour log the teachers' reasons for John's behaviour can also be discerned. There is a tendency amongst teachers, caught up in the pressures and maelstrom of large classes, to construe children with dyslexia in terms of laziness and lacking intelligence. They attribute the problem to constitutional (within the child) factors. In John's case, explanations for his behaviour seemed much broader and damning. He was considered to be behaving in such ways 'out of mischief', because he was 'obviously showing off', in 'an awkward frame of mind' and because he was 'obviously trying to make me cross'. One statement even suggested that John punched another child 'for no reason at all'! Kelly would have keeled over sideways. Behaviour, however perplexing to us, Kelly argued, must make sense to the child. They do not act in a vacuum. By considering this in regard to the sociality corollary it might be inferred that the relationship between John and his teachers was bereft of mutual understanding. Neither seemed able to construe the other's construction process, leaving their relationship lacking in rapport. As Bannister and Fransella (1986) suggested, if we cannot understand a child, that is we cannot construe his constructions, then we may indeed *do* things to him, but it cannot be presumed that we *relate* to him.

The behaviour log was also awash with predictions. Almost invariably, however, John's teachers appeared to have their predictions invalidated. They couldn't quite anticipate how their own attempts to relate to John would be received. Here are a few examples. Asking John to do his work led to point blank refusal, stomping across the classroom, but also to occasions of sustained compliance. Telling John to do his work led to point blank refusal but also disruptiveness. Confrontation made things worse but, just occasionally, John did alter his behaviour after a stern word. Finally, acknowledging his efforts positively 'obviously provided comfort' but then again praising his efforts sometimes led John to feel embarrassed and deface his own composition. Many of the teachers' predictions about John were therefore at sea. Kelly might have understood the teachers' predicament in terms of both anxiety (John became increasingly more difficult for them to understand in their pedagogic system of constructs) and hostility. Although recognising that John was becoming increasingly difficult to anticipate and manage, the teachers persisted in their efforts (Kellyan hostility) to construe John in ways they were familiar with. Whilst John rattled around an increasingly untenable system of constructs his teachers found themselves, rather than modifying their way of viewing John, encapsulating him within a series of pre-emptive and negative characteristics.

The police had a much more direct way of discovering if John understood the difference between right and wrong. In true Kellyan spirit they asked him. Following the charge of murder it was fairly predictable that John might respond to questions concerning wrongness with 'Don't go on high stuff and don't chuck stuff off'. What was perhaps less predictable was John's silence when asked if there was anything else wrong. To further direct prompts about whether stealing and telling lies were wrong, John said 'Yeah'. The paucity of John's replies reflect not an intention to obstruct but a staggering indication of the improbability that he construed events in terms of their rightness and wrongness. Here was a matter of imposing legal construing on to a child's version of events.

In listening to John talk about his and other children's behaviour, his superordinate construing seemed never to be in terms of right and wrong. Rather, John described behaviours in terms of fun, good, bad and those 'you get done for'. He had mentioned to the police that it was fun being bad and not fun being good. Fun for John was equated with playing, messing about, being cheeky, fighting, getting into trouble and being bad. He had a reasonably encyclopaedic view of being bad, but apart from being boring, being good was very poorly elaborated. Fransella (1972) has argued that individuals resist behaving in ways (being good for John) when their construing about that behaviour is only partially elaborated. In contrast behaving badly for John served to validate his version of himself. As Kelly intimated the way we construe determines the way we act.

In order that an understanding of John's superordinate construing of behaviour might be gathered, he was asked to sort a set of behaviours under three categories: fun (in contrast to good); wrong (in contrast to right); and ones you get done for (a phrase John had used in reference to law-breaking behaviour). *Table 7.2* presents the results of this

Table 7.2 Categorisation of behaviour

Behaviour	Fun	Wrong	Get done for
Being cheeky			✔
Calling names		✔	
Showing off		✔	
Telling lies		✔	
Fighting			✔
Messing about	✔		
Getting others into trouble		✔	
Talking in class		✔	
Stealing			✔
Bunking off school		✔	
Swearing		✔	
Damaging other people's things			✔
Hurting others			✔
Playing tricks on others		✔	
Breaking into places			✔
Throwing stones at others		✔	
Joyriding			✔
Housebreaking			✔
Vandalism			✔
Throwing stones off motorway bridges		✔	
Shoplifting		✔	

exercise which John completed without difficulty. He employed the wrong—right construct with discrimination, allocating eleven behaviours to this category. The closest behaviours to the one John had been charged with – throwing stones and throwing stuff off motorway bridges – were placed in this category of wrong. They were, however, not seen to be activities like joyriding and vandalism which John saw as breaking the law. It might therefore be contended that John was able to make a distinction between right and wrong, and indeed between wrong and seriously wrong (things you get done for) but that his actions on the roof that day (given he was unaware of the possible consequences) was not construed by John to be seriously wrong.

Intriguingly this inference bears a close correspondence to Gitta Sereny's (1995) conclusion about Mary Bell, the 10-year-old girl, found guilty in 1968 for the murder of two young boys in Newcastle. Because there seemed no reason for her to commit such iniquitous deeds, she was construed as an evil, freakish and monstrous child. However Sereny's careful study of the events concludes with the possibility that 'death, 'murder' and 'killing' had a different connotation for the girl than it had for other people. Basically for Mary, 'all of it had been a game – in the sense that an experiment can be a game for children – a grisly game, but a game nevertheless'.

Self image

John, it seemed, construed much of what he did it terms of being fun and bad. Kelly would contend that his actions were an expression of his construing and that they were essentially means of testing out his predictions and ultimately of how he saw himself. With this in mind, John was invited to complete two scales which would hopefully tap his sense of self – the Self Image Profile (Butler 1994, 1996) and the Harter (1985) 'What I am like' scale. The analysis of both these scales told a very similar story, and the attraction of both scales is that different aspects of self can be discerned. *Table 7.3* illustrates John's completed Self Image Profile and *Table 7.4* presents a summary of the Harter scale.

John had an extremely positive view of himself as a sportsperson. He was also very content with his appearance, apart from not liking curls in his hair. John also showed satisfaction in his kindness, helpfulness, honesty and what Harter described as general self worth.

The realms of self construing where John expressed dissatisfaction included his behaviour, schoolwork and social relationships. John's view of self appeared both discriminating and sophisticated. He acknowledged his struggle to master school work, recognised a concern about his behaviour and doing things he knew he shouldn't, and finally he demonstrated a profound unease about his ability to get along with others.

Social relationships

Dyslexia seems to alienate a child from others. John's view of himself contains a theme about loneliness and the wish for more friends.

Table 7.3 John's Self Image Profile

How would you describe yourself?	Not 0	1	2	3	4	5	Very 6
Kind						▨	
Make friends easily			▨				
Well liked	▨						
Good fun							▨
Lots of energy							▨
Helpful							▨
Honest					▨		
Good at sport							▨
~~Intelligent~~/smart ~~Dresses smartly~~*							▨
Like the way I look	▨						
Feel different from others		▨					
Lazy	▨						
Lonely							▨
Stubborn	▨						
Moody			▨				
Always in trouble							▨
Shy	▨						
Cheeky	▨						
Argue a lot	▨						
Bad tempered		▨					
Get bored easily							▨
Good at school work	▨						

*John understood the word 'smart' to mean 'dresses smartly'.

Poignantly the behaviour log at school makes many references to John's rejection by his peer group. *Table 7.5* provides some examples of how the teachers described John's behaviour in relation to classmates and how in turn they reacted to John. This portrayal points an unwavering finger at John as the source of trouble. It captures the teachers' feeling

Table 7.4 Results of the Harter 'What I am like' scale

School work	Appearance
Worry about whether I can do it	Happy with how I look
Slow at school work	Happy with my height and weight
Forget what I learn	Like my body the way it is
Don't do well at classwork	Like the way I look
Trouble figuring answers	Wished I looked different**
Just as smart as others*	Good looking
Total 11	Total 20
Social	Behaviour
Hard to make friends	Don't like the way I behave
Not many friends	Usually do the right thing
Like to have more friends	Act in ways I know I'm supposed to
Do things by myself	Get in trouble for things I do
Wished more people liked me	Do things I know I shouldn't
Popular	Find it hard to behave
Total 11	Total 14
Sport	General self esteem
Do well at all sports	Unhappy with myself**
Good at sport	Don't like the way I'm leading my life
Could do any sport	Happy with myself
Better than others at sport	Like how I am
Like to play rather than watch	Happy with the way I am
Good at new games	Way I do things is fine
Total 23	Total 19

*Smart for John meant being dressed smartly, not intelligent, as Harter intended it to mean. **John expressed a dislike for the curls in his hair.

of John being the creator of other children's discomfort and their ultimate rejection of him.

John's actions might be seen as validating his view of himself – they confirmed to him his academic inadequacy, his behavioural non-conformity and social alienation. However failure to play 'a social role' with others at school seems to have encouraged John to gravitate towards others outside of school who survived on what might be called the fringes of socially acceptable behaviour. Being a 'misfit' within one social domain (school) may have fostered the search for relationships where he could play a social role; where he could be understood by others; where his 'socially inappropriate behaviour' could not only be validated but elaborated. In such ways his incompetence could be transformed into an asset. So John, outside of school, sought friendships with other boys who were similarly in trouble. With a group of like-minded individuals John could conduct behavioural experiments – acting in antisocial ways – with a fair degree of anticipation that his efforts would be applauded and gain social acceptance.

Table 7.5 Some comments from the behaviour log which illustrate John's reported effect on classmates (names changed to preserve confidentiality)

Makes Billy show off
Sabotaged Darren's drawing
Class became noisy, having been excited by John
Called several people's mums a fat bitch, silly cow, fat slag
Tried to push others off grassy mound
Enticed others but no-one joined in
Other children asked me to send John to another class
Telling tales – the whole of the class atmosphere changed
Calls others rude names
Mocked others, upsetting them
Others disturbed by John's language and behaviour
Children complained about John
Prevents others from working
No child is impressed by John's antics
Other children swore – John's behaviour is apparently affecting one or two others
Tried to incite others
Class became high due to John's behaviour

In an attempt to understand how John perceived himself in relation to the other two boys who were on the roof with him, he was asked to undertake a ranking exercise. The names of the three boys involved – John, Alan and Carl – were written on separate cards and John was asked to place them in rank order against a set of activities. The results of this stab at understanding John's social role are illustrated in *Table 7.6.*

Table 7.6 John's ranking of the three boys against social activities

Social activity	Rank		
	1	*2*	*3*
Who's best at football?	Alan		
Who gets into most trouble?	Alan	Carl	John
Who's good at schoolwork?			
Who gets teased most?	John	Carl	Alan
Who gets his own way?	Alan		
Who messes about at school?	Carl	Alan	John
Who bullies others?	Alan		
Who worries most?	Carl		
Who gets upset?	Carl		
Who dares others to do things?	Alan		
Who gets into fights?	Alan		
Who is most bad tempered?	Alan		
Who gets bored?	Carl	John	
Who gets others into trouble?	Alan		

Fascinatingly, John declined to place any of the three boys alongside 'good at school work'. A perceived commonality was their abject failure to meet schools' expectations. Carl, the youngest of the three, was seen as the one most likely to become emotionally upset. Alan on the other hand was perceived by John to be the leader of the group (getting his own way) and the one to assert his power and domination over the other two through bullying, fighting and getting others into trouble. John ranked himself first on only one aspect, perceiving himself to be the victim of teasing. He went on to describe how Alan would bully, punch and steal things off him in order to make him do as Alan wanted. John claimed Alan was the instigator that morning, asserting that 'When we were playing that day, Alan said he were going to batter me if I didn't go up on the roof with him'. John claimed it was Alan's idea to 'play on the roof, throw stuff off, mess about and get into trouble'. John's acceptance within the group was therefore dependent on assuaging and currying favour with Alan. Even amongst his kindred spirit continued approval was threatened. John was possibly faced with the need to engage in ever more extreme acts in order to maintain 'credit', validate the antisocial aspect of his self construing and hold on to what he felt was a somewhat tenuous but fundamentally important relationship. Taken in this context, the act of tipping the cement block from the roof may have made perfect sense to John. It was an extension of previous acts which served to further define the notion of himself as a non-conformist troublemaker coupled with a prediction that such behaviour would foster a greater acceptance of other like-minded individuals, notably Alan.

The ironic tragedy in terms of social invalidation happened a few hours after the incident when, in police custody, John learnt that both his compatriots, as it were to save their own necks, turned against him. They claimed to have told John not to push the boulder from the roof. Ultimate rejection.

What appears legally to be a reasonably straightforward task of determining if John, at the time, knew that what he was doing was seriously wrong, turns out psychologically to be a somewhat thorny issue. There would seem to be little doubt that John knew he was engaged in behaviour that would probably get him into trouble. Indeed his very self identity was built on the notion that he was a trouble-maker, and his acts and misdemeanours served to validate this. If we act in ways governed by our self construing, then it might be argued that John had little choice but to act in such troublesome ways. Interestingly a Kellyan position would predict that having committed the act, John would not feel necessarily guilty because he was merely acting in a way he expected of himself. Guilt, according to personal construct theory, occurs when we discover ourselves acting in ways we would not have predicted of ourselves. The problem of 'fitting' a legal definition of wrongness on to John's actions is particularly illuminating, given that John 'naturally' construed events in terms of fun and getting into trouble *versus* being good, compared to the legal construct of wrong *versus* right. If John did not construe events in the manner proposed by the legal system, how would he be expected to know about wrongness? Getting into trouble, yes – indeed he was a connoisseur of this – but knowing it was wrong, well that's a different ball game.

To further compound the problem is the notion of acting in a way that might be described as seriously wrong. The prosecution has to demonstrate this in order to counter the presumption of *doli incapax*. The incompatibility of construing – John's construction of fun/getting into trouble *versus* the legal definition of wrong – still infiltrates and complicates the reasoning at this level. However there are some additional legal constructs which might be held up to compare how John's act measures against them. These include the idea of intent *versus* accident; preplanned *versus* an exception; and whether John considered the implications of his actions *versus* a consideration of only the moment in time. The legal definition focuses on an appreciation of what harm the behaviour might do to a victim, whereas it would seem John's focus and actions were directed more towards himself (seeking validation of his self image) and towards his compatriots (seeking to secure social allegiance with Alan).

Further 'expert witnesses' were asked by the prosecution and defence. Two saw John and another two commented on the reports. All concurred essentially with these initial findings. Disappointingly none of the reports was heard in court because of a pre-trial agreement between prosecution and defence. During the trial John appeared disinterested in the proceedings, frequently occupying himself in drawing pictures. After a trial lasting 4 days, the jury considered the evidence for 55 minutes and then delivered its verdict of guilty.

Postscript

Some might find themselves feeling uneasy about the foregoing account, perhaps a hint of the proverbial do-gooder's inclination to blame anybody but the little devil who threw the brick in the first place. Taking the argument further we might consider that the analysis excuses, rather than explains, some fundamentally inexcusable behaviour. What happens to the sense of personal responsibility which is central to the moral education we aim to offer young people when even the perpetrators of crimes are perceived as victims?

'It's not my fault – look at my circumstances', may not be a plea to which many might be immediately sympathetic. Indeed if judgements in cases such as John's boil down to 'Whose side are you on?', we probably have little hesitation in empathising with the elderly victim and her family. As an afterthought we might even find ourselves harbouring suspicions that these psychologists might end up doing more harm than good when they muddy the judicial waters with their fancy jargon and faddish theories of child development! All these questions are worthy of further examination.

Children's culpability

In order to be blameworthy in the eyes of the law a young person has to be aware that their wrongdoing is wrong. Age is reckoned to be a rough indicator of whether a child is capable of making this sort of moral judgement in much the same way that the competence of a juvenile witness in court will be gauged in part by how old they are. However there will be appreciable variation within as well as between age bands, so the question of whether any particular youngster knowingly misbehaved needs to be individually assessed, especially when that person is considered to be on the chronological cusp of moral awareness, at between 10 and 14 years of age.

The social context in which a crime has been committed becomes evident when more than one person is implicated in the act. If, for example, a gang of teenagers engages in a delinquent activity such as vandalising a bus shelter, the issue of personal culpability might depend on the perceived seniority of an individual within the group. Were they older 'ring-leaders' or more junior followers who had 'fallen in with a bad crowd'? Where an adult is adjudged to have played a destructive role in fostering juvenile crime it is the adult rather than the child whom we hold responsible. We despise Fagin and sympathise with Oliver.

Indeed children's legislation is designed primarily to protect children from adults rather than the other way round. For example the key principle of the Children Act 1989 that decisions be taken in the best interest of the child applies equally whether the young person has committed an assault or been himself the victim of one. In fact young people who commit offences of the person against others have often been physically maltreated themselves.

Where does this brief consideration of social and developmental aspects of juvenile crime leave us in our understanding of the individual case? Take another example:

> Ben is a 10-year-old boy recently admitted to a residential child psychiatric hospital because of concerns that his highly sexualised

behaviour indicates that he has been abused within his family home. While living in the unit he makes suggestive remarks to female staff and fellow residents. This inappropriate behaviour rapidly escalates culminating in two sexual advances on a particularly vulnerable girl patient. At a rapidly convened case conference the young man is viewed by some parties as being in need of treatment (as he is displaying the very symptoms which led to his admission to hospital in the first place) while others see him as needing to be controlled (as he has become a significant danger to others). The mood of the meeting swings dramatically, sometimes seeing him as a patient, sometimes as a perpetrator, and fails to come to any clear conclusions on his future management.

Is there a correct way to make sense of this episode? Personal construct theory argues that the same event is open to a myriad of more or less useful interpretations. The meaning of an act is not self evident but comes from our attempts to understand. So we can choose to attribute blame to individual failings and locate the problem within the individual as when we invoke the idea of a person being inherently 'evil'. We can place greater importance on situational factors and recognise mitigating circumstances if we so wish. We may strive to get a grasp of the actor's motives in committing an offence. In essence we evolve our own personal theories to try to make sense of the puzzling activities of others. The classic courtroom confrontation offers but two stories to account for a particular episode, those told by the prosecution and the defence counsel respectively, but there are many other ways in which the tale can be told. However, it appears that the discomfort which deeds such as the sexual abuse and murder of children evoke in us makes it difficult to engage in circumspect consideration of alternative explanations. We are tempted to take up a position pre-emptively as if ours were the only view that any reasonable person could adopt. In so doing we risk forgetting that there are always other ways of construing, and fail to realise that our capacity to envisage alternatives is limited by the time we live in, the family we came from, and the very people we are.

Psychological theory in the courtroom

Legal decision-taking is a formidably challenging exercise. Judgements must be made which will have a major impact on the future lives of all concerned. Due process must be followed so that justice is administered impartially. All voices must be heard with equal respect. Furthermore, everything must be completed as quickly as possible. In essence, the pressure is on to sum up individuals and their circumstances with maximum efficiency. What psychological models are likely to be best suited to this task?

Legal judgements invariably include elements of retrospective analysis and prospective prediction. Evidence is heard and its significance weighed. The question of guilt likely needs to be addressed. Those passing sentence or making recommendations about future management try to anticipate the probable outcomes of various courses of action open to them. This time perspective colours the ways we understand other people's actions. Looking back, human behaviour appears convincingly predictable. The apparently smooth and inevitable life-courses depicted in biographies of the great and good imply they were always destined for glory. The glaring oversights of some hapless social worker who has gravely failed to protect a child at risk of serious injury seems unforgivable when it is 'perfectly obvious' they would be harmed. But 20/20 hindsight teases us with an illusory clarity. At 2.45 pm the perceptive punter will be able to explain the outcome of the 2.30 race with expert confidence. He will note the impact of the going, the benefits of a draw close to the rails and of course the classic breeding of the winner on the dam's side. However when applying these self-same canons of wisdom to name the horse that will win the 3.00 race, our expert's breezy certainty diminishes somewhat, and he begins to hedge his proverbial bets. A world that can look so reassuringly predictable in retrospect has the unnerving habit of appearing confusingly erratic when we peer in the opposite direction (Green 1993).

A second powerful influence of perspective on the way we make sense of behaviour depends, as alluded to earlier, on our position as participant in, or observer of, the action under analysis. It is a well-established principle of social psychology that folk tend to adopt markedly different schemes when explaining their own actions compared to the system they apply to make sense of the behaviour of others. We have a penchant for putting our own failings down to passing situational factors such as an 'off-day' or adverse circumstances. However when we offer an opinion on the likely causes of somebody else's misdemeanours we seem more inclined to evoke enduring constitutional explanations for their fallibility – they are 'a bad lot' or 'not really up to it' and so on.

An example from the classroom might be a young lad with reading problems who persuades himself that his difficulties stem from the fact that the book his teacher has provided is too boring for anyone to concentrate on for more than 2 minutes. His teacher's analysis of events may tend to emphasise the pupil's limited intellectual ability in other aspects of his school work and a pervasive negative attitude to learning that can come across as a truculent laziness. Evidently when the child identifies circumstances, rather than some generalised personality characteristic, as the cause of his reading problem he can approach a new book with his self esteem reasonably intact and with some hopes of a more successful outcome next time around.

Indeed the way we attribute blame when things go wrong in our lives is a key determinant in our ability to maintain morale in times of adversity. It is less immediately obvious why observers should prefer to invoke trait theories when explaining the misconduct of others. Maybe we need a robust classification system to help us to sort out the wheat from the chaff among our fellow citizens – particularly those we don't know too well. Perhaps we have a faith that the world is an inherently just place where bad people get their just deserts. Sometimes this psychological shorthand works well and enables us to see enduring patterns in another person's conduct of which they are unaware. On other occasions our need to sum up people simply and quickly drifts into the sort of harmful stereotyping on which racial prejudice thrives.

In summary therefore, as observers analysing retrospectively the misdeeds of young people in trouble with the law our 'common sense psychology' will incline us towards explanations that emphasise the lasting personality characteristics of the individual perpetrator. We consider criminal tendencies to be in his nature in some sense and see a constitutional basis for his antisocial conduct. We would also be encouraged to adopt this viewpoint by the prevailing political ideology in both the USA and the UK in official attitudes to juvenile crime.

Do we need professional psychologists to put us right? The British judiciary doesn't think so!

Turner rule

The Turner Rule is a principle by which a court can determine the admissibility of psychological evidence. It runs as follows:

> *If on the proven facts a judge or jury can form their own conclusions without help, then the opinion of an expert is unnecessary. In such a case if it is given dressed up in scientific jargon it may make judgement more difficult. The fact that an expert witness has impressive qualifications does not by that fact alone make his opinion on matters of human nature and behaviour within the limits of normality any more helpful than that of the jurors themselves: but there is a danger that they may think it does. (Quoted in MacKay and Coleman 1991.)*

So while a judge might be prepared to invite a psychiatrist to offer a professional opinion on the state of mind of someone acting violently under the influence of paranoid delusions, he may not take kindly to psychologists pronouncing on a matter as commonplace as misbehaving youngsters throwing stones at their elderly neighbours.

It is therefore necessary to make a convincing argument that the personal construct approach to understanding the actions of young men like John adds something useful to the untutored psychology that might otherwise be employed in deciding his fate (Green 1993).

The personal construct analysis described lays great store on getting the 'inside story' on events. It pays attention not just to the circumstances under which a crime was committed but more importantly examines the individual's construction of that situation – how he saw it at the time. It explores in depth the miscreant's view of himself and his behaviour. Furthermore personal construct psychology frames its proposals in the form of hypotheses on how things might be understood rather than drawing dogmatic conclusions that purport to say how things actually are. Three useful possibilities emerge from adopting this attitude to the problem of deciding what to do about John:

1. Although our estimates about the constancy of our own and others' behaviour across time and circumstances are often misguided we do not live in an entirely chaotic social world that is quite beyond our comprehension. The better we know people the more accurately we can predict their behaviour. That tautological assertion begs the question of what it means to know another person well. When we know not just where a person works and whom they work with but also know what they think about their job and the company they keep, we can begin to anticipate accurately their performance in post. If we can add to this understanding an awareness of their sense of self confidence in their role, how they see their strengths and weaknesses and whether work matters much in their scheme of things, we are likely to make even more informed guesses. So an appreciation of the personal construct system of an individual provides us with a great deal of evidence which will be pertinent to our efforts at predicting their future behaviour.

2. Kelly proposed in his 'sociality corollary' that our ability to play a social role with another person depends crucially on our ability to see the world through their eyes or 'construe their construction processes' in his phrasing. For those responsible for promoting the healthy development of children – parents, teachers, social workers – this seems an eminently desirable principle. The better we understand what makes a particular child tick, the more effectively we can help them. But it also follows that if our primary concern is to control a young person's behaviour to reprimand or punish them, this task will also be more successfully achieved if the parties involved appreciate each other perspectives. If, on the contrary, adult attempts to sort out troublesome children seem to them to be ill-informed and incomprehensible our good intentions may well be

frustrated. Punishment that makes no sense to a recipient who does not feel their voice has been heard cannot but be experienced as persecutory.

3. Everyone agrees that something must be done to deter delinquents. Quite what must be done is however far from certain. While advocates of simplistic penal policies may play to appreciative galleries in the public bar or at the party conference, in practice effective remedies to counter juvenile crime are hard to find. Depressingly high reconviction rates seem to follow all forms of custodial sentence for juvenile offenders, and psychological treatments for young people exhibiting antisocial behaviour have no track record of proven effectiveness. We have no option but to keep thinking creatively about ways to judge each individual case on its merits and personal construct theory at least offers us a framework within which to consider our alternatives.

Chapter 8

Children and illness

'Ill conceived ideas'

Children, like the rest of us, don't like feeling unwell. Their suffering is often amplified by their inexperience of illness. They don't have any articulated theories about the causes of their discomfort, and they cannot predict the future course of, for example, a common cold because they have been through that 'sort of thing' before. They might be utterly perplexed when their apparently caring parents pour vile-tasting liquids down their throats and announce that this odd-coloured 'medicine' is doing them good. Sometimes previously trusted doctors and nurses go even further and stick needles into them – to make them feel better! In short from the child's perspective, illness is both painful and incomprehensible (Wilkinson 1988).

It's not that children make no attempt to understand their sickness or the ill-health of others. Rather they evolve their own idiosyncratic theories to make sense of their suffering instead of adopting the official grown-up medical explanations of illness. Paediatric psychologists have sought to map the stages through which the young person's thinking about ill-health typically passes en route from utterly uncomprehending infant to relatively sophisticated adult (Bibace and Walsh 1980). Characteristically preschool children are limited to thinking about their world in pretty concrete terms and have only a few primitive ideas about cause and effect relationships.

When a youngster is ill they might invoke a magical explanation for their misfortune. A young man, described in an American journal article, who overhearing his doctors describing his condition as 'oedema' concluded he must have 'a demon in his belly' (Perrin and Gerrity 1981). Another basic line of reasoning might go along the lines that if I'm hurting this bad I must have done something really naughty to deserve it. However not only children choose to construe ill-health as punishment for misdeeds. The 'gay plague' analysis of AIDS shares the same fundamental assumption that this is a just world we live in and pains are not generally inflicted without good reason.

Giving appropriate explanations

The implications of this developmental stage approach to children's understanding of illness for the clinical management of young children's health care is that parents and medical staff are advised to frame their explanations of treatment in age-appropriate terms so that youngsters can assimilate ideas into their prevailing scheme of things. Such advice may seem banal, as anyone with a dash of common-sense would pitch their conversation with a 5-year-old on a different, less complex level than that they would employ with a 10-year-old.

However the Piagetian approach, as it is called, holds more subtle possibilities for effective communication with such children. When preparing a 6-year-old for hospital admission it is advisable to describe the process in very concrete terms – where the bed will be, what colour the nurses' uniforms are, who will stay in hospital with the child, and so forth. Such information, pitched at the child's level of understanding, can help the child immediately grasp a vision of what is to happen and be informed in their anticipations of an otherwise mysterious and frightening prospect.

By giving a child information in a form they can readily use, adults assist the young person's theory-building. If, on the other hand, a well-meaning parent offers a more abstract explanation of how the medical treatment will alleviate the child's suffering (for example a tonsillectomy) the odds are that the conversation will go 'over the child's head' and remain unprocessed and hence sadly unhelpful in preparing for the forthcoming experience.

The Piagetian approach also reminds adults that children's construing of illness is different from their own. In discussing a child's sickness with him or her, there is a need to know about children as well as illnesses.

A final teasing implication of this developmental stage approach is the description of a narrow band of knowing that lies beyond the child's existing level of understanding but before the point at which he or she is destined to be lost by the sophistication of an overly-complex argument – outside the youngster's grasp but within his reach to coin the poet's metaphor. If adults can construe the thinking of the young person they are counselling well enough to pitch their conversation in this transitional zone they may enable the child to accommodate their thinking to new information in a way that moves them a step or two further up the developmental ladder (Green 1982).

Coping with illness

Piaget's model is primarily a cognitive one. He argues that the developing child's ability to make sense of the world is fundamentally constrained by their level of brain maturation. There are in-built intellectual limits on their capacity to understand. However those working with sick children rapidly note differences in the attitudes as well as the abilities of their young charges. One way of categorizing the attitude a person adopts to their illness is to construe them as exhibiting a characteristic 'coping style'. The assumption is made that we all, from an early age, develop a preferred way of getting by when confronted with life's problems. Whatever the difficulty, it can be argued that an individual will adopt an almost automatic way of coping such that their attitude might be considered more a personality trait than a chosen strategy suited to particular circumstances.

Although psychologists have produced a number of systems for classifying coping styles, the limited literature examining sick children's construal of their illnesses eventually boils down to a straightforward continuum between those who actively seek out information about their disease on the one hand, and those who elect to 'switch off' and deliberately ignore their condition on the other (Kupst 1994).

This tendency to 'attend' or 'deny' puts quite contrary demands on carers. Do parents research suitable books or videos to enable their child to get better informed about an illness, or do they continue to live family life 'as normal' with no acknowledgement of their child's ill-health? By and large it appears young people who adopt an active coping style manage hospital admissions for surgery better than those who 'cross that bridge when they come to it'. They tend to experience less pre-admission anxiety, are more co-operative within hospital, and report less postoperative pain (Schultheis *et al.* 1987).

The following case vignette illustrates the disadvantages of adopting an 'I don't want to think about it' approach to a painful medical procedure:

> Cheryl is a 9-year-old girl recently diagnosed as suffering from leukaemia. She doesn't discuss her condition or its treatment at all within the family and is applauded for this 'stiff upper-lip' approach by her father who uses the same coping style himself. Cheryl gives every sign of carrying on regardless, her morale remaining high, and she deals with most aspects of her treatment regime with robust good humour. However a central element in her therapy involves regular infusion of drugs through a 'portacath' inserted just below her neck. Cheryl never mentions her feelings about this procedure but becomes very agitated and uncooperative at home when awaiting the ambulance that takes her to hospital on the 'portacath' day. When her turn for treatment comes she

resists efforts to help her keep control of the process (e.g. to say when the needle goes in) and kicks out and swears at her mum and the nursing staff who subsequently find themselves having to manhandle Cheryl to ensure she receives the treatment she needs to combat a life-threatening disease.

No one concerned gets any satisfaction from this sequence of events. Cheryl feels frightened and humiliated. Nursing staff are very uncomfortable at physically imposing treatment on an unwilling young patient. Cheryl's mother dreads these 'portacath' days on which she is subjected to abuse and assault from her daughter, but also helps hold her down while she screams in pain. However Cheryl point-blank refuses to discuss other ways of preparing for, or coping with, this evidently troubling component of her care.

At first sight it seems evident that Cheryl's dominant coping style of denial is equipping her poorly for managing a key aspect of her treatment. However, would it be desirable to try and turn her into an active coper, even if it were achievable? Would there be more therapeutic mileage in working with her preferred way of getting by when under stress (e.g. by distracting her in the clinic room) than challenging the only way she knows how to cope just when her very life is under threat?

A further uncertainty is added by the finding that patterns of coping might be determined by the situation as well as the person. Young cancer sufferers, for example, report a higher level of denial on 'coping style' questionnaires than members of matched control groups with other health disorders. Furthermore 'switching off' as a way of dealing with the overwhelming anxieties of discovering you have cancer is a more common way of coping directly after initial diagnosis, than at the later stages of treatment. Maybe, therefore, there is something natural and adaptive in Cheryl's attitude to her disease and its treatment.

The psychology of children with illness is not a psychology of abnormal children but of normal children reacting to a quite abnormal situation (Eiser 1990). It therefore makes sense to conduct research into the experiences of sick children who share the same diagnostic label and symptomatology, and must cope with common treatment regimes (for example children with diabetes who need to control their diet and receive daily injections of insulin).

Unique experience of illness

All these approaches to children's understanding of illness make sense. Without doubt it is important to consider the age and intellectual competence of the individual, their preferred coping style and the particular characteristics of their disease and its treatment. However, what is missing from these models is a way of appreciating the unique way in which each young person constructs their experience.

In Kelly's view there are external realities with which we have to contend in which ill-health can surely be numbered. However individuals do not all wrestle directly with the same objective challenges. They interpret their worlds. Thus some people's colds always seem worse than others! Hence sharing a diagnosis with another person gives no guarantee that their experiences of illness will be identical. Diagnostic labels probably mean a lot more in the doctor's construct system than in their patient's – or certainly mean something different to the two parties. Therefore it might be apposite to view sick children as 'unique protagonists each on their own unique journey' to use Phil Salmon's (1985) persuasive phrase.

Inevitably individual children's ways of understanding their predicament will be limited, perhaps by factors associated with their biological maturity, but also by the small but expanding repertoire of constructs that they have available to try to make sense of their lives. They will seek to make sense of illness in the same way they seek to make sense of other events they confront. They cannot consult a medical textbook to find out what's going on when they get ill. They have to work it out for themselves in their own idiosyncratic way.

Sometimes these 'childish' constructions are a source of amusement for adults and are portrayed as visible failures to understand. Personal construct psychology asserts that if only we could see things through the eyes of the individual child, their versions of what it means to be unwell would make perfect coherent sense. However, that is a very big 'if only'.

Understanding the child's version

Charlie's story gives an idea of how apparently 'senseless' actions of a sick adolescent can become comprehensible once we get access to the 'inside story':

> Charlie was a 13-year-old boy who had suffered since his birth from a congenital urinary problem. This meant that he was prone to infections which had a cumulatively deleterious effect on his health. Despite being old enough and apparently wise enough to appreciate the dangers he faced if he picked up infections, Charlie persistently took avoidable risks and ignored his parents' sound advice about wearing suitable clothing when going out in the cold and wet. He seemed to court illness by waiting for his school bus dressed in shirt-sleeves during a bleak Yorkshire winter. Charlie's exasperated parents couldn't decide whether he was stubborn or stupid.

Charlie didn't much enjoy his psychological consultations but he was able to produce a number of constructs to describe himself (such as 'likes football', 'gets called lazy' and so on). In an effort to discover which of these ideas mattered most to him Charlie completed a resistance-to-change grid (Hinkle 1965). First, all of his constructs were laid out on a sheet of paper with a preferred and unpreferred pole clearly marked (e.g. 'likes football' *versus* 'boring creep'). Then every construct was paired with every other construct and Charlie asked to answer the following unusual question:

- If you had to move from your present position on one of these two scales towards the end you like least, on which would you choose to stay put?

This exercise results in a league table of constructs from those on which the individual is relatively happy to move in their less prepared direction up to those on which they are most resistant to change. Hinkle argued that we resist change on our most 'superordinate' constructs - those that matter most to us as individuals. Top of Charlie's league table came a construct concerning his health ('feeling well' *versus* 'getting sick'), and one about feeling normal ('being just like everyone else' *versus* 'being different'). However it was the latter construct that was the more resistant to change. In other words if faced with a choice of being socially or physically handicapped Charlie would prefer sickness to the social stigma of standing out from the crowd. Hence if the other school hardmen eschewed warm winter clothing, so did he.

Sharing an understanding of construing

What are the therapeutic explanations of taking seriously Kelly's celebration of the uniqueness of individual experience for those charged with the care of sick youngsters? Maybe the clearest message is that as much attention should be paid to helping the doctor under-stand the child as is paid to trying to enable the child to understand the doctor. It is appropriate to think hard about the explanations given to young people about the medical treatment they receive. It is important that they find procedures and interventions predictable and to feel some sense of control over events. Where possible children should be helped to appreciate the motives of those who cause them discomfort.

As children grow older clinicians should also aspire to give them choices so they can give informed consent and enter a genuine collab-oration with their carers. It is important to achieve clarity in the explanations given to children and seek to be as transparent as possible in conveying our understanding of their illness and its treatment. In so doing the application of Kelly's sociality corollary is half way towards being achieved. At the risk of repetition this corollary states that '*To the extent that one person construes the construction processes of another, they may play a role in a social process involving the other person*'.

Health care is unarguably a social process. Personal construct analysis highlights a recognition that doctor–patient communication is a *two*-way traffic system. There is good sense in training health personnel to improve their broadcasting skills and educating patients, of whatever age, to be attentive receivers of important medical messages. But how should the views of children be conveyed in the other direction? Health professionals in training are required to parade their constructs about illness in public examination. They are tutored in how best to get their ideas across to patients.

In contrast, sick children have no comparable preparation for playing their part in a medical consultation. Few can, or will, articulate their views on their condition with any confidence, and so probably 'know' much more than they can easily tell. Most will have relied on a parent to represent their case to a doctor (a bit like a lawyer in the courtroom) and hence held only the most perfunctory of conversations directly with health care staff. It is therefore going to take a deal of time and invention if sick children are to be encouraged to relate their own stories of illness.

However it is likely to prove a worthwhile effort because the doctor who ignores their patient's perspective jeopardizes the effectiveness of treatment just as securely as the patient who ignores their doctor's advice. For example research with children who wet their beds (Butler *et al.* 1990) has indicated that an understanding of the meaning enuresis has for the particular child will both improve the accuracy of predictions of their probable response to treatment, and open up therapeutic avenues to enable the individual to consider some of the social and psychological implications of becoming dry.

Negotiating perspectives

The central tenet of personal construct theory is that there is no single veridical way of making sense of any event (including the phenomenon of ill health). There are a myriad of possible different theories and interpretations all of which may be judged more or less useful depending on the job to be done. The physician's job of 'treating illness' is different from the young patient's job of 'growing up with illness'. The manual needed to control symptoms differs from the map required to get on with life. Both tasks are crucial. Both construct systems need to be fitting to their purpose. So recognition and negotiation of a necessary difference in perspective is required for the business of effective health care to be completed.

The same principles apply within families. Parents, siblings, and sufferer have different jobs to do and need to evolve construct systems fitting to their respective responsibilities (Sloper and White 1996). You do not have to share another person's view of the world to get on with them, Kelly argues, but how successfully you can co-operate on any joint enterprise does depend on how well you can read and respect each other's scripts.

Commonality of construing

Acknowledging the uniqueness of individual experience does not deny the usefulness of classifying sick children according to their similarities so that the health resources they need can be most effectively organised. Kelly argued that this necessary grouping might as well be achieved by putting together individuals who share a common view of the world, as by aggregating individuals that are commonly viewed by the world.

Rather than categorise sick youngsters together according to diagnosis – children with asthma, sufferers from cystic fibrosis, those with enuresis and so forth – an alternative might be to bring together or consider groups of young patients with a particular coping style, such as those who seek to deny the implications of their illness, or those who become sensitive and vigilant about symptoms (e.g. Fritz and Overholser 1989). When young people who have taken part in group psychotherapy are asked what profited them most from their sessions together, a frequent reply is the sense that they are not alone in their thoughts and feelings – others hold similar views. So self-help groups or peer-tutoring arrangements (where an older child helps a younger partner learn to better understand his or her condition) take advantage not just of the similar circumstances with which a cluster of children are confronted but also some of the shared attitudes they are likely to adopt towards their predicament (Shute and Paton 1990). For example, a pair of adolescents with diabetes must both have to inject themselves with insulin on a regular daily basis, but might also both find themselves feeling highly resentful about the inflexibility of this regime and how it precludes them from 'hanging loose' like other teenagers.

Ill-health and identity

The development of an individual's sense of their unique identity is widely construed as the major psychological task of adolescence

(Erikson 1968). To achieve this goal successfully it has been suggested that the young person must negotiate an increasingly autonomous relationship from their parents, begin to define themselves as an adult through some productive work effort, and construe themselves as sexually mature in a physical and social sense. Ill-health may complicate all these aspirations.

If the developmental drives of adolescence usually have a centrifugal impact on the family system, illness is likely to exert a quite contrary pull on family members to stick together (Rolland 1987). The young person's physical condition may compel them to rely on their parents in a way that under other circumstances might not be considered age appropriate (in getting help with bathing for example). Parents' anxieties (that for example a teenager with diabetes may lose consciousness) may make 'letting go' of an adolescent son or daughter problematic for fear that this offspring will come to avoidable harm if left unsupervised.

Ill-health can confuse the developing individual's sense of their own sexuality. Sometimes a disease or its treatment will have a direct impact on growth and the timing of puberty (for example some cancer treatments). More commonly a young person who has experienced illness or injury has concerns about their physical attractiveness and may be very self-conscious about, for instance, their weight, or physique. Frequently ill-health places constraints on the opportunities young people have to mix with peers and engage in group activities such as sports or other leisure pursuits, and so the individual feels less socially prepared for the challenge of courtship. They don't feel ready in the sense that both their own sexuality and that of potential partners remains a mystery. It is, of course, arguable that uncertainty and discovery are intrinsic characteristics of all new relationships. That promise of excitement is why people choose to pursue fresh liaisons in the first place. However personal construct theory reminds us that while we may sometimes opt for the adventurous alternative through which our views of ourselves and other can be elaborated, we can also choose to stick with what we know and find predictable. Ill-health does not often bring out the bold explorer in any of us, whatever our ages.

Illness can have major vocational implications. Schooling may well be disrupted, so reducing the person's prospects of academic success. This may have a direct effect on grades achieved in public examinations and hence restrict access to further training opportunities (Madan-Swain and Brown 1991). More subtly, scholastic underachievement will influence the individual's emergent sense of competence and self-efficacy. Physical ill-health may also block a number of potential career routes. Poor eyesight, asthmatic reactions to dusty conditions, limited mobility and so on will all close off certain occupational possibilities. For young people with a life-threatening disease such as cystic fibrosis whose families dare not adopt a long-term perspective on adult life-plans, the issue of what job the child may want to do when they grow up just does not arise. For all these reasons the stepping-stone to adulthood that the first wage packet represents may prove beyond the easy reach of young people whose development has been complicated by significant experience of illness.

This analysis of the way in which ill-health can interfere with the process of identity development applies whether the individual has suffered from chronic illness from an early age, or is obliged to reconstruct their emergent sense of identity when experiencing major ill-health for the first time in adolescence. This task of re-definition is daunting at any point in a person's life (after a stroke in a late-middle age for example) but perhaps the teenager whose sense of identity remains plastic and somewhat confused anyway, has even more on their plate.

Two brief case examples illustrate how hard it can be for adolescents whose development has been compromised by ill-health to construct a satisfactory sense of self:

Neil has suffered from the unusual skin complaint epidermolysis bullosa (basically thin skin) throughout his life. At age 16 he can reflect poignantly on how growing up with chronic illness has stopped him from 'living out the other parts of my life'. He is socially anxious, friendless and highly self-critical, reserving his strongest condemnation for the person he is, rather than the condition he's got. He can be very hurtful and mocking towards his parents on whom he remains very reliant. Neil cannot walk very far unaided, needs assistance with the administration of some skin-care medication, and generally has a poorly developed capacity to look after himself (he won't shop independently, cannot make himself a meal, etc.). His troubled attitude towards his mother and father could be characterised as resentful dependence. He is taking some GCSEs but appears uncommitted to further education. He scoffs at the thought that any girl might be prepared to go out with him.

Steve was 17 when he suffered a closed head injury in a motor-cycle accident, after which he was hospitalized for over 8 months. Therefore he subsequently has a number of gross physical and psychological handicaps including hemiparesis and spasticity, slow slurred speech and pronounced sexual disinhibition. Before his accident Steve was an apprentice mechanic – an occupation he is no longer equipped to pursue. Twelve months after receiving the injuries that have palpably ended his motor-cycling days for ever, he continues to describe himself as 'a biker through and through'. However he also reflects sadly that most of the time he can barely recognise himself in the way he feels and reacts. He is lost within his own skin. Steve's parents want to encourage their previously free-wheeling son to resume an independent social life, but dread the consequences of Steve's disinhibited impulses for his own, and other people's safety.

What can a personal construct approach offer to young people in such dire straits? To paraphrase Kelly 'its not what your illness or injury has made of you that matters, but what you make of it'. There are realities of treatment regimes and painful symptomatology that need to be confronted, but when Kelly asserted that everything which exists can be reconstrued, he meant everything. What does it mean personally to discover you have diabetes? What implications does having 'petit mal' epilepsy have for how you construe yourself? These are questions to be personally considered and reconsidered. There is no 'that's it' finality imposed by medical diagnosis.

Personal construct psychology emphasises the importance of developing a schema to allow the individual to anticipate events. One consequence of the appropriate mourning for 'what might have been' (in Steve's bike fantasies for example) is that the person with health problems may have a very well-articulated sense of the person they could/should have become.

For constructive adaptation to the world they actually live in, they need to create a similarly detailed map of their current possibilities. Just like Fransella's group of stutterers who needed help to think of themselves as fluent speakers before they could make best use of technical speech therapy advice (Fransella 1972), young people who are unwell may need reminding that sickness does not write your life script for you. History is not destiny. Part of the strong sense of stigma that sick children frequently report stems from a feeling that they have become *nothing but* a diabetic, a cystic, a haemophiliac or whatever.

The sociologist Goffman famously subtitled his treatise on stigma, '*The management of spoiled identity*' (Goffman 1963). The optimistic message of personal construct theory is that 'spoiled' is a construct open to revision, not an immutable life sentence. However our views of ourselves are socially as well as personally constructed and children's self concepts are substantially influenced by their understandings of how other people react to them. So it is important for health professionals to ensure that they see the person beyond the diagnosis. The risks involved in children failing to acknowledge the consequences of their illnesses might easily be recognised, such as when an adolescent with diabetes undertakes a bout of prolonged exercise without considering the impact on their blood sugar levels.

But there are parallel dangers when adults construe young people as nothing but a diagnostic category. Even in a condition such as autism that so impairs the social development of the individual, the concerned outsider who pays close attention and listens carefully can get to appreciate the singular characteristics of each evolving person. The neurologist Oliver Sacks (1995) displays just such an attitude of respectful curiosity towards the patients he meets and describes in his books and films. You always get the sense of being introduced to an individual, rather than encountering a syndrome. If medical consultations never go beyond diagnostic labels we should perhaps be concerned for the psychological wellbeing of the doctor as well as for their patients. As Kelly wryly observed, 'hardening of the categories' can be an awfully debilitating condition!

References

Bannister, D. (1962) The nature and measurement of schizophrenic thought disorder. *Journal of Mental Science*, **108**, 825–842.

Bannister, D. (1963) The genesis of schizophrenic thought disorder: A serial invalidation hypothesis. *British Journal of Psychiatry*, **109**, 680–686.

Bannister, D. (1983) The experience of self. Paper presented at the 5th International Congress in Personal Construct Psychology, Boston. Unpublished.

Bannister, D. and Agnew, J. (1977) The child's construing of self. In J. Coles and A. Landfield (eds.) *Nebraska Symposium on Motivation 1976*. Lincoln, NE: University of Nebraska Press.

Bannister, D. and Fransella, F. (1986) *Inquiring Man: The Psychology of Personal Constructs* (3rd ed.). London: Croom Helm.

Bibace, R. and Walsh, M.E. (1980) Development of children's concepts of illness. *Pediatrics*, **66**, 912–917.

Bronowski, J. (1973) *The Ascent of Man*. London: BBC Publications.

Butler, R.J. (1985) Towards an understanding of childhood difficulties. In N. Beail (ed.) *Repertory Grid Technique and Personal Constructs*. London: Croom Helm.

Butler, R.J. (1994) *Nocturnal Enuresis: The Child's Experience*. Oxford: Butterworth Heinemann.

Butler, R.J. (1996) *Sports Psychology in Action*. Oxford: Butterworth Heinemann.

Butler, R.J. and Hardy, L. (1992) The performance profile; theory and application. *Sport Psychologist*, **6**, 253–264.

Butler, R.J., Redfern, E.J. and Forsythe, W.I. (1990) The child's construing of nocturnal enuresis: A method of enquiry and prediction of outcome. *Journal of Child Psychology and Psychiatry*, **31**, 447–454.

Butler, R.J., Redfern, E.J. and Holland, P. (1994) Children's notions about enuresis and the implications for treatment. *Scandinavian Journal of Urology and Nephrology*, Suppl. **163**, 39–48.

Butler, R.J., Hiley, E. and Roberts, G. (1996) *Parental Intolerance: Recognising the Signs; Assessing the Degree; Finding Solutions*. London: Ferring.

Butler, R.J., Hiley, E., Roberts, G. *et al.* (in preparation) An investigation of the impact of nocturnal enuresis on children's self construing.

Dalton, P. and Dunnett, G. (1992) *A Psychology for Living: Personal Construct Theory for Professionals and Clients.* Chichester: Wiley.

Donaldson, M. (1984) *Children's Minds.* London: Fontana.

Edwards, B. (1988) *Drawing on the Artist Within.* Glasgow: Fontana.

Eiser, C. (1990) *Chronic Childhood Disease: An Introduction to Psychological Theory and Research.* Cambridge: Cambridge University Press.

Elliott, C.D. (1983) *British Ability Scales.* Windsor: NFER-Nelson.

Epting, F.R. (1984) *Personal Construct Counselling and Psychotherapy.* Chichester: Wiley.

Epting, F.R. (1988) Journeying into the personal constructs of children. *International Journal of Personal Construct Psychology,* 1, 53–61.

Erikson, E.H. (1968) *Identity, Youth and Crisis.* New York: Norton.

Fransella, F. (1972) *Personal Change and Reconstruction: Research on a Treatment of Stuttering.* London: Academic Press.

Fransella, F. (1995) *George Kelly.* London: Sage.

Fransella, F. and Bannister, D. (1977) *A Manual for Repertory Grid Technique.* London: Academic Press.

Fransella, F. and Dalton, P. (1990) *Personal Construct Counselling in Action.* London: Sage.

Fritz, G.K. and Overholser, J.C. (1989) Patterns of response to childhood asthma. *Psychosomatic Medicine,* 51, 347–355.

Glover, J. (1991) *I: The Philosophy and Psychology of Personal Identity.* London: Penguin.

Goffman, E. (1963) *Stigma: Notes on the Management of Spoiled Identity.* New York: Prentice-Hall.

Green, D. (1982) Moral development and the therapeutic community. *International Journal of Therapeutic Communities,* 3, 209–217.

Green, D. (1993) Constructs in the courtroom. Paper presented at the Xth International Personal Construct Congress. Townsville, Australia.

Green, D. (1997) An experiment in fixed role therapy. *Clinical Child Psychology and Psychiatry,* 2, 553–564.

Harter, S. (1978) Pleasure derived from challenge and the effects of receiving grades on children's difficulty level choices. *Child Development,* 49, 788–799.

Harter, S. (1985) *Manual for the Self Perception Profile for Children.* Denver, CO: University of Denver.

Hartley, R. (1986) 'Imagine you're clever'. *Journal of Child Psychology and Psychiatry,* 27, 383–398.

Hinkle, D. (1965) The change of personal constructs from the viewpoint of a theory of construct implications. Unpublished PhD Thesis, Ohio State University.

Hughes, M. (1986) *Children and Number: Difficulties in Learning Mathematics*. Oxford: Basil Blackwell.

Jackson, S.R. (1988) Self Characterisation: Dimensions of Meaning. In F. Fransella and L. Thomas (eds) *Experimenting with Personal Construct Psychology*. London: Routledge Kegan Paul, pp. 223–229.

Jackson, S.R. and Bannister, D. (1985) Growing into self. In D. Bannister (ed.) *Issues and Approaches in Personal Construct Theory*. London: Academic Press.

James, W. (1892) *Psychology: The Briefer Course*. New York: Holt.

Kelly, G. (1955) *The Psychology of Personal Constructs* (Vols I and II). New York: Norton.

Kelly, G. (1969a) Sin and psychotherapy. In B. Maher (ed.) *Clinical Psychology and Personality; The Selected Papers of George Kelly*. New York: Wiley.

Kelly, G. (1969b) The autobiography of a theory. In B. Maher (ed.) *Clinical Psychology and Personality: Selected Papers of George Kelly*. New York: Wiley.

Kelly, G. (1970) Behaviour is an experiment. In D. Bannister (ed.) *Perspectives in Personal Construct Theory*. London: Academic Press.

Kelly, G. (1980) A psychology of the optimum man. In A.W. Landfield and L.M. Leitner (eds.) *Personal Construct Psychology: Psychotherapy and Personality*. New York: Wiley.

Kupst, M.J. (1994) Coping with paediatric cancer: Theoretical and research perspectives. In D.J. Bearson and R.K. Mulhearn (eds.) *Pediatric Psycho-oncology: Psychological Perspectives on Children with Cancer*. Oxford: Oxford University Press.

Mackay, R.D. and Coleman, A.M. (1991) Excluding expert witness: A tale of ordinary folk and common experience. *General Law Review*, 800–810.

Madan-Swain, A. and Brown, R.T. (1991) Cognitive and psychological sequelae for children with acute lymphocytic leukaemia and their families. *Clinical Psychology Review*, 11, 267–294.

Mair, J.M.M. (1977a) Metaphors for living. In A.W. Landfield (ed.) *Nebraska Symposium on Motivation 1976*. Lincoln, Nebraska: University of Nebraska Press.

Mair, J.M.M. (1977b) The community of self. In D. Bannister (ed.) *New Perspectives in Personal Construct Theory*. London: Academic Press.

Mancuso, J.C. and Adams-Webber, J. (eds.) (1982) *The Construing Person*. New York: Praeger.

McCoy, M.M. (1977) A reconstruction of emotion. In D. Bannister (ed.) *New Perspectives in Personal Construct Theory.* London: Academic Press.

Neimeyer, R. and Harter, S. (1988) Facilitating individual change. In G. Dunnett (ed.) *Working with People: Clinical Uses of Personal Construct Psychology.* London: Routledge.

Perrin, E.C. and Gerrity, P.S. (1981) There's a demon in your belly: Children's understanding of illness. *Pediatrics,* **67**, 841–849.

Ravenette, T. (1977) Personal construct theory: An approach to the psychological investigation of children and young people. In D. Bannister (ed.) *New Perspectives in Personal Construct Theory.* London: Academic Press.

Ravenette, T. (1980) The exploration of consciousness: Personal construct interventions with children. In A.W. Landfield and L.M. Leitner (eds.) *Personal Construct Psychology: Psychotherapy and Personality.* New York: Wiley.

Ravenette, T. (1988) Personal construct psychology in the practice of an educational psychologist. In G. Dunnett (ed.) *Working with People: Clinical Uses of Personal Construct Psychology.* London: Routledge.

Rolland, J.S. (1987) Chronic Illness and the life cycle: A conceptual framework. *Family Process,* **26**, 203–221.

Ronen, T. (1996) Constructivist therapy with traumatised children. *Journal of Constructivist Psychology,* **9**, 139–156.

Rowe, D. (1983) *Depression: The Way Out of Your Prison.* London: Routledge and Kegan Paul.

Rutter, M. and Yule, W. (1975) The concept of specific reading retardation. *Journal of Child Psychology and Psychiatry,* **16**, 181–197.

Rutter, M. and Yule, W. (1979) Reading difficulties. In M. Rutter and L. Hersov (eds.) *Child Psychiatry: Modern Approaches.* Oxford: Blackwell, pp. 556–580.

Sacks, O. (1995) *An Anthropologist on Mars: Seven Paradoxical Tales.* London: Picador.

Salmon, P. (1970) A psychology of personal growth. In D. Bannister (ed.) *Perspectives in Personal Construct Theory.* London: Academic Press.

Salmon, P. (1976) Grid measures with child subjects. In P. Slater (ed.) *The Measurement of Intrapersonal Space by Grid Technique* (Vol. 1). Chichester: Wiley.

Salmon, P. (1985) *Living in Time.* London: Dent.

Salmon, P. (1995) *Psychology in the Classroom: Reconstructing Teachers and Learners.* London: Cassell.

Schultheis, K., Peterson, L. and Selby, V. (1987) Preparation for stressful medical procedures and person + treatment interactions. *Clinical Psychology Review,* **7**, 329–352.

Sereny, G. (1995) *The Case of Mary Bell: a Portrait of a Child who Murdered*. London: Pimlico.

Shute, R. and Paton, D. (1990) Childhood illness – the child as helper. In H.C. Foot, M.J. Morgan and R. Shute (eds.) *Children Helping Children*. London: Wiley.

Sloper, P. and While, D. (1996) Risk factors in the adjustment of siblings of children with cancer. *Journal of Child Psychology and Psychiatry*, **37**, 597–607.

Smith, D.J. (1994) *The Sleep of Reason: The James Bulger Case*. London: Century.

Tschudi, F. (1977) Loaded and honest questions: A construct theory view of symptoms and therapy. In D. Bannister (ed.) *New Perspectives in Personal Construct Theory*. London: Academic Press.

Wilkinson, S.R. (1988) *The Child's World of Illness*. Cambridge: Cambridge University Press.

Wing, L. (1981) Asperger's syndrome: A clinical account. *Psychological Medicine*, **11**, 115–129.

Winter, D.A. (1992) *Personal Construct Psychology in Clinical Practice: Theory, Research and Application*. London: Routledge.

Index